“The Hand of God”

"The Hand of God"

The Story of John Keating and the Power of Love

Mike Keating and Judy Keating

Writer's Showcase
San Jose New York Lincoln Shanghai

"The Hand of God"
The Story of John Keating and the Power of Love

Writer's Showcase
an imprint of iUniverse.com, Inc.

For information address:
iUniverse.com, Inc.
5220 S 16th, Ste. 200
Lincoln, NE 68512
www.iuniverse.com

ISBN: 0-595-15224-4

Printed in the United States of America

To Melynda
With all our love and gratitude

Contents

Preface

We have long discussed the writing of this story but never seemed to find the time. When we finally did sit down to write, it was an emotional experience because it brought back many long suppressed feelings. The driving force to write the story was the grandchildren. We wanted them to know the story of their father's accident, his courage and recovery, and the power of love.

The title is significant and meaningful to the family because it seemed to be not only a visual reminder but also an emotional well-spring of hope and faith during the entire ordeal. *The Hand of God* is a sculpture by Carl Milles (1875–1955), Sweden's most famous sculptor. The work is a study in creative and divine force and is located in Millesgarden on the island of Lidingo, northeast of Stockholm, not too far from where we lived. It stands in the sculpture garden near his villa beside the sea. It was a constant reminder to all of us of His grace.

The quotations used throughout the text are from conversations and the letters we received. The letters as they appear in the book have been corrected for spelling and some punctuation. In addition, they have been edited to remove very personal and private matters, which are not germane to the story and could only potentially embarrass those involved. For the most part, the letters are reproduced as originally written.

Acknowledgements

We wish to thank the many people who took the time to write letters, to visit, to call, and to be there for us when we needed you. You are the ones to whom we owe the largest debt of gratitude. Those of you who were part of this experience know who you are. Please accept our deepest appreciation.

To those friends who read and commented on the preliminary draft of the book, we are grateful. Thanks to all of you—Harold and Yvonne Lathan, Leah Salter, Chuck and Joyce Kaysing, Dick Pivetz, and Gloria Simons.

We also wish to thank Lew Simons and Paula Mathis for their editorial guidance, Brian Belsterling for his assistance with the graphics, Jan Gagnor for her typing support, and Salli Marks for her technical editing.

Our family remains our most precious gift. Thank you, Joanne, for your patience and understanding; and John, for your encouragement and collaboration. Both were key to the success of this project. Without a doubt, John's wife Melynda and their children have been John's greatest blessing.

We are constantly inspired by the love of our entire family. They have made our dreams come true.

Introduction

Montgomery, Alabama
April 9, 2000

Dear Lane, Asa, and Gabriel,

Not long ago, Dee and Papa began writing the story of your Dad's accident and subsequent recovery. We felt it was an interesting and inspiring story, which you would want to hear.

It was a difficult time for the entire family. We survived primarily because of the courage and determination of your Dad. He was an inspiration to all and a hero to many, some of whom he never even met. In the hospital in Uppsala, he was a legend known simply as "the American."

Your Dad was given a task rarely imposed upon one so young, and he met the challenge with outstanding courage and exemplary determination. Papa has seen war and the courage of men in the face of death. He has seen men suffer, their bodies torn and souls scorched in the crucibles of pain, and he has seen men die. One often associates courage with war, but your father's courage was no less than that of any soldier.

Since the accident, we have been asked countless times: "How did you survive? How did you cope with such a tragedy?" The answers are not easy. First of all, we felt that the only viable option as a family was to cope. We, in a sense, had no other options. If your Dad was fighting for his life, we were going to be there with all the love and support we could muster. We are sure that our attitude was a reflection of the love we have within the family and the love of those close to us. Certainly the support we received from family, friends, associates, and people we did not even know was also a major factor. They furnished the intangible strengths we so desperately needed. They provided the fuel to keep our emotional gas tanks full.

In the book, *An Illustrated History of St. Albans School,* The Reverend Mark Mullin, the Headmaster, wrote:

> Friendships forged at St. Albans have a way of becoming strong and durable. Ten months after he graduated, a member of the Class of 1980 was involved in an extremely serious accident. He probably had not thought a great deal about sense of community while a student, but he wrote me from his hospital bed:
>
> "Please give my thanks and my love to all the students at St. Albans. I realize, after this accident, that my years at St. Albans created something—a kind of loving bond between my classmates, my instructors, and the student body. I am making a fantastic recovery, and the doctors are quite amazed. I know my speed of recovery is directly related to your prayers and concern. I'll make it through, I know, because of the strength I'm gaining from my friends."
>
> That young man had learned something worth knowing.

That young man was your Dad! There is actually no way we can explain the importance of the support of family and friends and the significance of their letters. One had to experience it; had to read the letters themselves. Therefore, we wish to share the story and the letters with you.

Love,
Dee & Papa

Chapter One

The Accident (April 8–9, 1981)

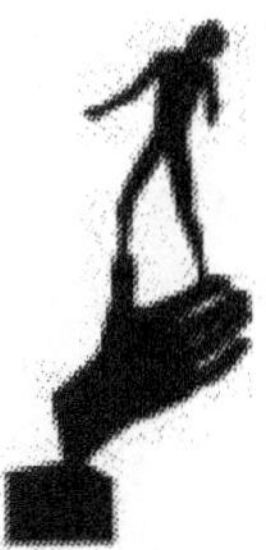

*　　　*　　　*

I wish we could have the future back.

—*Joanne Keating*

*　　　*　　　*

The day had been absolutely beautiful—clear and cold—and the skiing that morning was excellent. After lunch John had entertained the children in the lodge with his hand puppet, Animal, of the Muppets. There was no language barrier among the many nationalities gathered as

Animal opened and closed his mouth, growled and raised his eyebrows. The children laughed joyfully as Animal went through his routine. They had seen John skiing earlier with Animal hanging tightly around his neck.

That afternoon, John and Animal continued to delight the children on the slopes. The children would point with glee and tell their parents about the American and his friend Animal. When the skiing ended for the day, the children followed John and Animal into the lodge like the Pied Piper.

Nineteen year-old John and his 18-year-old sister Joanne were with their parents, Mike and Judy Keating, at a ski resort in Storlien, Sweden, located approximately 350 miles northwest of Stockholm. The Keatings were on assignment to the American Embassy in Stockholm where Mike, a colonel in the United States Air Force, was the Defense Attaché and Air Attaché (DATT). The Swedish International Office of the Ministry of Defense (Fo/INT), the office with which all foreign military attachés were accredited, had just completed their annual Winter Trip for the attachés. The orientation provided an opportunity to experience the environment in which the Swedish military had to operate in defense of the country in this cold, mountainous, and desolate region of northern Sweden.

The Winter Trip began with a day of briefings about the defense of this region given by the responsible Military Command. Attachés were outfitted with the equipment used by these highly talented ski-troopers, including skis and boots. For the next two days, the attachés learned to use, as best they could, the equipment—especially the skis. The accomplished skiers assisted the novices, and after a couple of days of training, the group set out on a five-day trek in the barren wasteland of northern Sweden. The trek's final destination was the ski resort at Storlien where the families of the attachés met the weary travelers for a respite and downhill skiing. It was here on April 8, 1981 the Keating family found themselves enjoying Sweden's picturesque mountains.

After dinner, there was dancing. Joanne had danced with Admiral Calle Algernon and was quite pleased with herself. She had enjoyed the evening but now, like almost everyone else, was ready to retire in preparation for another day of skiing. Joanne was sharing a room with Caroline Puntan, the daughter of Rosemary and James Puntan, the British Military Attaché. Their son Tim was sharing a room with John. As Joanne and her parents headed for their rooms, John, Caroline, Tim and some other young adults headed for the hotel's disco to continue the party.

Around midnight, the group left the disco and headed back toward the main lodge. The evening was storybook perfect. The sky was clear, the air fresh, and the light from the moon and stars created an iridescent glow on the snowy landscape. It was one of those moments of absolute beauty that defies description. It can only be experienced as a defining moment, the punctuation to a perfect day. As the group passed the small but quaint train station, someone suggested, "I bet the view from on top of one of those train cars is unbelievable!"

"Yeah! Let's have a look," came a response.

As the group moved towards one of the tank cars, John said, "I'm going up to see the view!" and he crushed out his cigarette. Someone threw a snowball. John retaliated. He reached down, made another snowball, and began climbing the ladder on the railroad car.

Halfway up, he threw the snowball at the group below, and as he neared the top, his thoughts shifted to the incredible grandeur of the view. The contrast of the dark sky with its sparkling stars and the glowing snow covered mountains extending up into the sky as if they were reaching up to God. He was awe-struck and yelled to the others to join him.

He innocently waved to his companions, completely unaware of the potentially deadly overhead electrical power line used by the Swedish railroads. His left hand hit the 16,000-volt power line.

The night lit up as if a giant flashbulb had gone off. John's body was highlighted by the electrical power, and he fell. It was a surreal picture with John falling as if in slow motion. His friends gasped in horror as John fell, hitting the ground with a sickening thud. Everyone froze; no one believed what they had just seen. Individually and collectively they waited to wake up from this nightmare, but nothing happened. As their senses began to return, Caroline ran to John's side and knelt down beside him.

"John!" she yelled. "John, are you all right?"

There was no response. John laid there, his eyes staring upward. Finally his eyes focused on Caroline and he moaned. Caroline knew that he was alive, but for how long? Smoke rose from his body like the early morning mist off a lake. The pungent smell of charred flesh was nauseating.

Someone yelled, "I'll get a doctor. There is one on call at the hotel."

Tim had moved beside his sister as she talked to John and said, "I'll go get his parents."

"Good. I'll stay with John. Hurry!" she replied.

John briefly raised his head and looked at his charred hand, his body still smoking. He waited to catch his breath. *Relax,* he thought. *Wait for the breath. Wait. Be patient.*

It seemed to be taking too long. He knew he was hurt, but not how badly. The pain eased, becoming distant, unreal. He thought of his Mom and Dad, and then Tim and Caroline, and finally the $20.00 he owed Dave Singer, a St. Albans classmate. He felt himself begin to drift away from his body and towards a brilliant light source. The pain had ceased, and he found himself floating above the accident scene looking down. He saw Caroline kneeling beside him and heard her calling to him.

I've got to get back down there and let her know I'm all right, he thought. Suddenly he felt his lungs fill with the cold night air. He began to call out Caroline's name and as he did, he returned to his body. So did the pain. The sound of Caroline's voice kept him conscious and alive. He knew if he could hear Caroline and feel the pain, he was alive and had a chance. He fought to maintain consciousness.

"John," he heard Caroline call.

"Where's my hat?" he heard himself say. "I lost my cowboy hat."

"We'll find it for you, John," Caroline said reassuringly. "You just relax; we'll get it for you."

"It hurts, Caroline. Oh! It hurts!"

"I know, John. We've gone for help. Tim has gone for your Mom and Dad."

"I can't lose my hat. Please find it for me."

* * *

There was a loud pounding on the door. Mike rolled over and Judy poked him saying, "Someone's at the door."

"Colonel Keating, Colonel Keating!" said a voice loudly as the pounding continued unabated.

"I'm coming," Mike said as he found the light switch and made his way to the door. *Who the devil could that be at this hour?* he thought as he opened the door.

Tim stood there with another young man, both looking as if they had seen a ghost and completely out of breath.

"John's been hurt," Tim gasped. "He burned his hand and fell off a tank car. Caroline is with him. Come quick. We'll take you there."

The Keatings quickly dressed as Tim and his companion paced in the hall. "Tim!" called Colonel Keating after both he and Judy had dressed and were lacing up their boots. Tim came back into the room.

"What happened?" Mike asked.

"John burned his hand and fell off a railroad tank car he had climbed," Tim explained. "They have summoned a doctor," he added. "Come quickly. It's just at the bottom of the hill."

The group moved quickly through the hotel. As they hit the cold night air, the shock of the freezing temperature underscored the fact that this was not a nightmare but reality. They hurried down the hill toward the railroad station.

The seriousness of the events began to take hold as they approached John, his body still smoldering. A few bystanders had come from the disco to see what was going on but remained at a respectable distance.

"The doctor is on his way," someone said. "Should be here shortly."

Someone else volunteered, "There is a stretcher at the hotel. I'll get a truck and bring it down so we can move him into the station."

John was conscious and recognized his parents but was in extreme pain. "I'm sorry, Mom," he said.

"That's all right, John," she replied.

"I'm so sorry. Please forgive me," he repeated.

Judy stayed with John while his father returned to the hotel to involve the Swedish military. He called Major Ove Hall's room and told him John had been in a serious accident, was burned quite badly, and he needed his assistance. Mike waited in the lobby for Ove, and when he and Major Ingemar Pedersson arrived, they set out for the station. Both Ove and Ingemar were assigned to Fo/INT and were the project officers for the Winter Trip.

They reached the station as Dr. Hemberg was arriving. With help from some volunteers, they moved John onto the stretcher and into the warmth of the station where the doctor began to assess the injuries. When he cut away John's jacket above his charred hand to view the extent of the burn, there was a gasp from the crowd. Above John's wrist, there was nothing but bone. No flesh whatsoever. The sight of a skeletal arm with a charred, black hand on the end of it rapidly thinned the crowd. The doctor immediately cut the other jacket sleeve open and began an IV.

John asked his father if he could remove his boots because they felt uncomfortable. Both his parents had been members of the National Ski Patrol and were experienced at removing ski boots from an injured person even if the leg was broken. Mike began to remove the boots.

The right one was no problem; but, as he attempted to remove the left one, it felt like the flesh was coming off with the boot, so he ceased.

"Gonna have to leave the left one on, John. Your foot seems a little swollen. Maybe later when some of the swelling goes down a bit."

"Okay," John replied.

Mike then walked outside and sat on the steps, his head in his hands, wanting to cry—but no tears would come. He had no way to release his emotions; he felt tremendous fatigue. It was like when one is extremely tired but can't sleep. *Maybe later when some of the hurt goes away,* he thought. Judy came up, sat beside him, and put her arm around him giving him reassurance and comfort. He cried then, but the emotional release he wanted and needed was not there, and the pressure continued to build.

* * *

Ove Hall approached the Keatings as they sat on the steps to brief them on the arrangements to have John, accompanied by Dr. Hemborg, transported by ambulance to the hospital in Ostersund. Mike, Judy, and Ove would follow in a taxi, which had been summoned. Judy asked if she could accompany John in the ambulance, and arrangements were made for her to do so. The follow-on stage of the evacuation would be for John to be flown to the Uppsala University Hospital Burn Center, which was the Burn Center for all of Scandinavia.

Not long after they had departed Storlien, John was extremely uncomfortable and was experiencing intense pain. He moaned, "I can't make it, Mom. I can't make it!"

"Yes you can, John. We will make it!" she responded.

The doctor determined that John was in too much pain to continue overland since his vital signs were weakening. They were now racing against the clock; John needed to be transported to Ostersund as fast as possible. Dr. Hemborg had the ambulance driver radio ahead to a small dispensary and arrange for a helicopter to meet them. John was moved into the dispensary to await the helicopter. Although he was quite uncomfortable, his vital signs improved with the rest.

A short while later, the distinct sound of helicopter blades was heard as the pilots made their approach into the helipad. John was loaded onto the helicopter and, as it lifted off, the windblast of the helicopter in the sub-zero temperatures was not felt by his parents, numbed by the shock of the events of the last several hours. As the lights of the helicopter faded into the night, they stood there in silence wondering if they would ever again see their son alive.

The moment was broken by Ove Hall calling the Keatings to the waiting taxi to continue their trip to Ostersund. They arrived at the hospital a little over an hour later and were met by a doctor who introduced herself as Dr. Elizabeth Axelsson.

"We have stabilized John and prepared him for his flight to Uppsala. His vital signs are good, and we have induced a medical coma. At the present time, the airport in Uppsala is experiencing heavy fog so we will be unable to transport him until the fog lifts. Hopefully, just after dawn," she explained.

"I have examined John and briefed the Burn Center on his injuries. They are expecting him and have a burn team awaiting his arrival," she added.

She asked them if they had any questions or if she could get them anything; they shook their heads no. There was no sense of time for the couple as they sat comforting each other. Ove Hall was attentive but respected their privacy as the couple quietly sat there. Finally, as dawn broke, Ove informed the Keatings that the fog still had the airport closed but they were expecting it to lift within the next hour or two. Mike took the opportunity to call the American Embassy.

"American Embassy!" said the voice of the Marine security guard.

"This is Colonel Keating. Is Chief Nowery in yet?"

"No, sir."

"I need to get a message to him as soon as he comes through the door."

"Yes, sir. I can take care of that."

"Good. Tell Chief Nowery that the DATT's son has been seriously injured in an electrical accident. He is presently in the emergency room at the hospital in Ostersund, and that we will be leaving here shortly by air ambulance for the University Hospital in Uppsala. I will call him when we get to Uppsala."

Sergeant Rush read back the message and, as a final thought, added, "Good luck, sir."

"Thanks."

Chief Master Sergeant George Nowery was the Operations Coordinator for the Defense Attaché Office (DAO). He was an extremely talented and resourceful individual with vast experience in dealing with the Embassy bureaucracy, having come to Stockholm from the Embassy in Vienna.

Ove Hall suggested that Mike accompany John to Uppsala in the aircraft while he and Judy returned to Storlien in the taxi. Judy could pack their belongings and pick up Joanne while Fo/INT made arrangements for her and Joanne to travel back to Stockholm via commercial air. Mike asked Ove if they would also contact Commander Greg Gushaw, the Assistant U.S. Naval Attaché, to inform him of Judy and Joanne's arrival time and Judy's desire to travel directly to Uppsala.

Commander Gushaw was a first-rate officer and individual who spoke fluent Swedish. His reporting was insightful and thorough. He and his lovely wife Carol had established close ties with the Swedish Navy that were unparalleled. High-ranking Swedish officers frequently complimented Mike on Greg's talent and demeanor. In addition, Greg and Carol were extremely popular within the attaché community.

Dr. Axelsson told the Keatings that the fog was lifting and the air ambulance would be waiting for them when they arrived at the airport. As John was being loaded into the ambulance, the couple embraced and went their separate ways. The aircraft lifted off at approximately 7:00 a.m. for the 1 hour and 15-minute flight to Uppsala. Mike sat in a jump seat next to John, staring down into his expressionless face. *He's out of pain now,* Mike thought. As he watched him breathe, the tears began to flow uncontrollably, lasting the better part of the flight.

* * *

After the ambulance had departed Storlien, Tim and Caroline made their way back to the lodge, still in a state of shock. They went directly to their parents' room and awakened them. They recounted the events of the tragic accident as their parents listened in horror and disbelief. When they had finished, Rosemary instructed her daughter to try to get some rest in their room and she would go to Caroline's room and be there when Joanne awoke. Tim went back to his room and began packing John's things.

Judy and Ove drove back to Storlien in silence. When they arrived, Judy went immediately to her room. On her way, she met Rosemary in the hall.

"Joanne knows there has been an accident but does not know the seriousness of it," Rosemary said. "She's in her room. I'll bring her to you."

"Thanks."

Joanne is a learning disabled child who has suffered from epileptic seizures since the age of four. The seizures have never been fully controlled despite the use of multiple anti-convulsive regimens.

Judy explained to Joanne that her brother had been injured in an electrical accident, and the extent and seriousness of his injuries were still unknown. She revealed it was life threatening, but prayed he was going to be okay.

"We need to pack all your things because we have to fly back to Stockholm. John and Dad are on their way to a hospital in Uppsala. We will be leaving here in about 30 minutes."

Rosemary helped Joanne collect her things, and Judy stuffed their belongings into suitcases and bags. Ove Hall returned, saying that they would bring the luggage back with them in a couple of days, including skis, boots, and so forth.

As the three were leaving the hotel, Judy turned to Rosemary and handed her a lift ticket. "Please give my lift ticket to Tom Yamasaki. It's good for the next couple of days."

Colonel Tom Yamasaki, the Japanese Military Attaché, was a friendly and outgoing individual who was skiing for the first time. During the trek, he had been paired with Mike who had helped him learn the basics of skiing.

Joanne, Judy, and Ove Hall then immediately departed for the airport. There was no time to see or talk to anyone. They had packed and departed in a matter of minutes.

Ove Hall and Ingemar Pedersson had been coordinating the operation and keeping their people up to date on what was going on. At breakfast word had spread that John had been seriously injured and evacuated to Uppsala. As one of the mothers was explaining to her young child that Animal's friend had been injured and had to go to the hospital, the child looked up into her mother's face and with an expression of great concern asked, "Did Animal get hurt too?"

* * *

As the aircraft taxied to the ramp where the ambulance stood waiting, Mike's thoughts drifted to his own parents. *Mom would have been 72 today. God, how I miss them!*

The aircraft stopped and, as the engines shut down, the door opened and medical personnel carefully removed John from the aircraft. Mike disembarked and an ambulance attendant motioned him to the front seat. Before he even had a chance to thank the flight crew, they were driving away. But he noticed the crew wave to him and give him a thumbs-up. This simple but meaningful gesture meant so much!

As the ambulance rolled into the emergency room entrance, medical personnel came rushing out, instructing the driver to deliver the patient directly to the burn unit. They arrived a minute or two later at the rear entrance of the main hospital. From there they boarded an elevator that took them to the fifth floor. Exiting the elevator, they crossed a small hallway towards some double doors, which opened to the group. The attendant pushed the door control button and they entered what appeared to be some type of air lock chamber. The doors closed behind them. Mike thought, *John, we finally made it. I hope we are in time.* Almost immediately the double doors at the far end of the chamber opened. There stood half a dozen people dressed in scrubs, including masks and rubber gloves. They came forward and took the gurney as one of the doctors approached Mike.

"Please come with me," he said.

Mike followed him into a small waiting room where he offered him a seat. "I'm Dr. Hedlund and I would like to brief you on exactly what we'll be doing to your son for the next few hours," he said in excellent English.

"Thank you!" Mike replied anxiously.

"First we will take cultures from John in order to study the bacteria present on his body. In about a week to ten days, John will be fighting infection, so we are collecting bacteria samples now and studying them so we better know how to fight the infection, which is inevitable," Dr. Hedlund explained.

"Infection is a major obstacle to survival for burn victims," he said pointedly.

The doctor explained that there exists a grace period of a day or two in the treatment of a severely burned patient. During that period the patient may be transported, but afterwards the odds of survival begin to rapidly diminish. He spoke frankly, relating that Brooke Army Hospital in San Antonio, Texas, was one of the best facilities in the world for the treatment of burn victims, and if we wished to have John transferred there, the decision would have to be made sometime within the next several hours.

"Is the treatment any different in the U.S. from what it is here in Sweden?" Mike asked.

"No," the doctor answered. "The treatment protocol is the same."

"Are you as good as Brooke?" Mike asked.

Dr. Hedlund smiled. "Yes. I think we are. In fact, our doctors have visited Brooke, and many of their doctors have visited us here in Uppsala. There would be no difference in the treatment."

"I tend to feel that John would be better off here because the family unit would remain intact, and that can be a major factor in any recovery process," Mike replied.

"We don't have to make that decision right this minute as we will be doing a medical assessment first," Dr. Hedlund said.

After a short pause, he continued, "After we take the cultures, we will bathe John in an antibiotic solution and then attempt to assess the extent of his injuries. This will take about an hour or two, so if you wish to go out to get something to eat or just walk around, please feel free. I'll be back to discuss where we stand after I examine John."

"When will you amputate his arm?" Mike asked.

"Let's not get ahead of ourselves," the doctor cautioned.

"Have you seen John's arm?"

"No."

"I have."

* * *

As Mike exited the hospital, a blast of cold air hit him—the first sensation he'd felt since he left the resort hotel some nine hours earlier. He walked aimlessly down the hill towards the center of town.

He had no sense of time or distance. His mind was racing through the events of the last several hours. His thoughts jumped from past remembrances to shattered future dreams. He felt tired but could not rest. He felt the helplessness when one has nowhere to turn but to God. He asked only for the strength to do his best in the ordeal unfolding about him. He felt the despair of being alone and thought of Judy and Joanne. Suddenly, he no longer felt alone. He was sure at that moment Judy was thinking of him and they were experiencing some type of shared togetherness. He recalled moments in Vietnam when he had experienced similar instances even though they were half a world apart. Finally, he checked his watch and started briskly back towards the hospital.

At a small sundry shop he bought a pocket notebook. He wanted to be able to tell Judy everything the doctors said, overlooking nothing.

* * *

Dr. Hedlund returned to the waiting room. Mike rose to meet him, anticipating his medical assessment.

"We need to operate on John's leg to improve the blood circulation and assess the damage. We'll use X-rays to study the circulation. We are going to keep him unconscious for a couple of days, keep him on a respirator, and hook him up to a kidney machine to clean the protein and potassium out of his blood. There is a danger to his heart if the potassium gets too high." There was a note of gravity and caution in Dr. Hedlund's voice.

He paused briefly and then continued carefully, "Our initial assessment is we need to amputate his arm. An amputation of the leg is uncertain at present as we need to determine where and if there is any circulation in the leg. The damage to his internal organs, especially his heart and kidneys, is unknown at this time. They are prepping him for surgery right now, and I'll be going to the operating room when we finish. Amputations are planned for tomorrow. We can arrange for you to spend the night here in the hospital if you so desire."

"Thank you, but no," Mike replied flatly. "We live in Djursholm, only about an hour's drive from here, so I think his mother and I will just go home. But thank you for the offer."

Mike still felt emotionally numb, but the milieu of the burn unit and the professionalism of Dr. Hedlund gave him a sense of relief and confidence that John was in very capable hands. Although terribly fatigued, he sensed a ray of hope for the first time since the accident.

Dr. Hedlund left, and Mike picked up the phone to call the American Embassy.

"Defense Attaché Office," Sandy Collins said.

"Sandy, this is Colonel Keating. Let me talk to Chief Nowery, please."

"Yes, sir. How are you doing? We're all praying for you," Sandy said.

"Thanks. I'm doing okay, I guess."

"Hello, Colonel Keating. This is George. I got your message. I've sent out a casualty report and USAFE has a KC-135 standing by to fly John to Brooke. How is John doing?"

"He's holding his own right now. They are scheduled to operate shortly."

"Great. Commander and Mrs. Gushaw, along with Tord, will meet Mrs. Keating and Joanne at Bromma. Fo/INT called with the flight number, ETA, and an update of what they knew about the accident. Tord will drive them to Uppsala in the Mercedes with Commander Gushaw following in the Volvo. Tord can leave the Mercedes there for you and Mrs. Keating and drive the Gushaws back in the Volvo. They should arrive in Uppsala by early afternoon."

Tord Robinson was a Swedish national who took care of the DAO's four official cars. He was also Mike's driver and functioned as a handyman, the DAO's jack-of-all-trades. He had been with the American Embassy since the late forties and was a man of great character and loyalty. He had been in the Swedish merchant marines in his youth and had suffered a crushing injury to his head. The injury had diminished his intellect, but he was man of substance, character, and deep feelings—a loyal and trusted friend who had an attachment to the American military as if they were family. He was an outspoken advocate of freedom and the American way and was as anti-communist as he was pro-American. He had an athletic, muscular body and, even in his 60's, could probably handle himself admirably in any type of street fight. His large, calloused hands could be as gentle as he himself could be compassionate. His greatest enjoyment was in helping others.

Mike briefed Chief Nowery on the contents of the conversation he had just had with Dr. Hedlund.

* * *

The landing at Bromma was smooth. As they taxied in, Judy's only thoughts were of John. It was hard to believe that just 24 hours earlier they had been skiing and having a good time. The whole family was together for this outing, and everyone had been looking forward to this quality family time. It was going to be a time for growing closer.

Tragedy also has a way of fostering growth and closeness, as the days ahead would attest.

The feeling of being alone magnifies the feeling of helplessness, and as Judy moved towards the terminal and saw Carol and Greg Gushaw and Tord standing there, her feelings of being alone seemed to lessen. A sense of relief came over her as she and Joanne were greeted with hugs and tears. They moved quickly to the waiting vehicles. Tord drove Judy, Joanne, and Carol, while Greg followed in the other car. The trip to Uppsala was quiet, but the two mothers shared a strong and nurturing compassion. The Gushaws suggested that Joanne return to Stockholm with them and spend the night with their two girls, Eve and Paige. Judy agreed, but remembered that Carol was going to leave for a trip to Finland with a group of ladies from the Embassy the following evening and insisted Carol not alter her plans. Carol reluctantly agreed, knowing that they shared a bond of mutual respect and admiration—one that would last a lifetime, and upon which Judy could rely and gain strength in the emotionally-charged days and months ahead.

* * *

Judy moved swiftly across the waiting room in the burn unit into the arms of her husband. They sat down holding each other. Mike spoke softly to her about John's situation as Dr. Hedlund had related it to him. They both agreed the idea of one of them accompanying John to San Antonio was unbearable. Medically speaking, John was in extremely capable hands, and they felt the emotional strength needed for all of them to overcome this tragedy would begin with the family remaining together. It would be synergistic. They tried to reassure Joanne, even though she was somewhat unaware of the seriousness of the accident. They felt relieved that she was going home with the Gushaws. After the group left with Tord, Judy and Mike sat together in silence, reeling from the shock left by the events of the past 15 hours.

Dr. Hedlund appeared at the door and entered the room. Mike introduced him to Judy and the three sat down.

"John is doing fine," the doctor began. "He is on the ventilator and has been hooked up to a kidney machine. His vital signs are strong and he has youth on his side. There is always a potential risk that he will go into shock, but the initial treatment provided by the emergency unit was excellent. The starting of an IV so promptly may have saved his life. We have every hope."

"Will you be operating again tomorrow?" Judy asked.

"Yes. We will be removing his arm tomorrow. How much, we don't know, but it will be substantial. We also will be amputating his leg, probably about mid-calf. We want, if at all possible, to make the amputation below the knee. We also will be doing some more X-ray studies to check on blood circulation."

A young man entered the room and Dr. Hedlund introduced him as Bosse, the chief nurse for ward 79-A, the burn unit. Dr. Hedlund said that Bosse would take us back to John's room shortly as John was returning from the operating room. The doctor then excused himself, and as he was leaving Mike spoke up, "Doctor, we have decided not to have John moved to San Antonio."

"Fine. We'll do our best." And the doctor was gone.

Bosse was a very pleasant young man but appeared to be a little young to be the chief nurse in this very specialized ward. Age aside, the Keatings quickly found him to be very adept and exceptionally well qualified for that position. He gave the couple the ward's telephone number and told them to call any time. He also assured the two that he would call them if there were any changes in John's condition.

Bosse then led the couple out of the waiting room and down a very wide hall towards John's room. As they entered his suite, they came first into a small anteroom where everyone washed their hands and donned a hospital gown, mask, and cap. Bosse explained that everyone who enters the room must go through this ritual for the first couple of days because of the threat of infection.

Mike and Judy could see their son tucked in among numerous machines, with tubes running all over the place and monitoring devices blinking and displaying data. A nurse sat there observing the monitoring devices. A brief feeling of relief came over them knowing that John had successfully made it this far. As they entered the room, they could hear the breathing machine's rhythmic swishing and the beeping of the monitoring devices. The welcome sounds of life interrupted the awkward silence. John looked peaceful but they could perceive the stress their son's body had endured. They stood there in silence.

The clock on the wall showed 7:45 p.m.—a mere 20 hours since the accident.

Bosse broke the silence.

"He's showing a lot of fight. He's scheduled for surgery tomorrow morning at 11:00. Please feel free to call me anytime for any reason. If I'm not here, any of the nurses will help you."

As the couple left the room and reentered the anteroom, tears choked their thoughts again. They silently stuffed their gowns, masks, and caps into the trash receptacle.

Walking down the hall, their eyes met those of the Swedish nurses who worked ward 79-A. Their compassion and understanding was evident. This was just a prelude to the impact these very special people would have upon their lives. For the nurses' part, they were about to embark on a memorable journey with a young man who became known simply as "the American."

* * *

But gallantry comes in unexpected ways, even unrecognized by the hero, who does what he does because that's the way he is.

—Ted Eagles

* * *

Deputy Chief of Mission & Chargé
Embassy of the United States of America
Stockholm, Sweden
April 9, 1981

Dear Judy and Mike,

There is no way to tell you with what sense of shock and grief Jeanne and I, and all members of the Embassy family, learned of the latest and grievous disaster to your family.

I simply want you to know that John is in our thoughts and prayers, and that we stand ready to help whenever and in whatever way you can signal us.

Sincerely,
Bill

*　　　*　　　*

P 101600Z APR 1981
FM DIA WASHINGTON DC//DR//
TO USDAO STOCKHOLM
UNCLAS
PERSONAL FOR COL AND MRS MICHAEL KEATING, DEFENSE ATTACHE, SWEDEN, FROM LT GEN TIGH, DIRECTOR DIA

"MIKE,

I CANNOT TELL YOU HOW BADLY WE FEEL AT THE NEWS OF YOUR SON'S ACCIDENT. PLEASE KNOW OUR PRAYERS ARE WITH YOU ALL. IF THERE IS ANYTHING AT ALL I CAN DO TO HELP, PLEASE ASK.

GENE"

*　　　*　　　*

Jacquie Barcilon
Lidongo, Sweden

April 10, 1981

Dear Judy,
What can I say to you and Mike other than to assure you of our friendship and help?

Perhaps when we—and I say we because both Robert and I feel we are in this with you having suffered the same sort of thing two years ago—are in calmer waters you will call us—we can talk and together get through the worst time.

We would very much like to visit John when this is permitted and again perhaps you could let us know when this is possible.

Dear Judy, God bless, and please know, even though it is little comfort at the moment that you and Mike are very much in our thoughts.

With our love,
Robert & Jacquie

*　　　*　　　*

Chapter Two

The Critical Days (April 10–19, 1981)

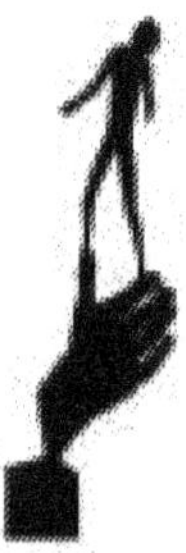

*　　*　　*

Having your constant love and care is strength to him and his fight to recover is sustaining power for you.

—*Mary Cronin*

*　　*　　*

The Keatings awoke from a deep sleep a bit disoriented, but as they lay there, the events of the previous day crystallized in their minds. They felt physically spent and emotionally drained.

"I'll call Uppsala," Mike said as he swung out of bed.

"I'll fix something to eat," Judy replied.

"Hello, this is Colonel Keating. May I please speak to Bosse?"

"Bosse is not on duty now. This is Elizabeth. John went down to surgery about an hour ago. He had a good night. His vital signs are good. The operation is scheduled to last three to four hours."

"He's doing okay?" Mike asked, desperately seeking reassurance.

"Yes," Elizabeth said. "He's doing very well. He won't be out of surgery until early this afternoon if you want to come up to see him then."

"Good," he said. "We'll be up about two."

Mike dressed, grabbed a bite to eat, cleaned up the kitchen, and wandered into the living room. He could hear music from the musical *Jesus Christ Superstar* playing, and when he walked into the den, he found Judy sitting quietly on the floor sobbing.

Running through her mind was the image of her healthy 19-year old athletic son as he was before the accident, and the fact that as she sat there he was undergoing life-saving amputations. *Amputation,* the thought of the word made her shudder.

Would he survive? And in what condition? she pondered.

Mike knelt down putting his arm around her and whispered, "I love you." They sat there together in silence just listening to the music. Finally, it was time to head for Uppsala.

Prior to leaving their house, Judy called Carol to check on Joanne.

"She's doing fine," Carol said. "You and Mike go on up to Uppsala and don't worry about her. She and the girls are having a great time. How's John?"

"They are operating on him now, and we're headed back up there to speak with the doctors after the surgery. There is nothing we can really do there, so we'll probably be heading back late this afternoon. We'll swing by and pick up Joanne."

"She's welcome to stay here with Greg and the girls."

"Thanks, but she needs to be with us tonight and hear that John is going to be okay. I only pray he will be."

"I understand."

"Have a great trip to Finland."

"Thanks."

* * *

Fight like hell, buddy. You know as well as everybody and anybody that you're worth it.

—Tom Liddy

* * *

The trip to Uppsala was quiet as the events of the previous day raced through their minds. As they approached the hospital, the feelings of dread and concern closed in around them. They parked the car, hurried inside, up the elevator, through the air lock, and into the Burn Unit. They went in silence, each with their own thoughts. One of the nurses recognized them, smiled and spoke.

"I'm Elizabeth. We spoke earlier. John is still in surgery but should be coming back soon. You may wish to wait here in the waiting room."

Swedish women are world renowned for their beauty and the female nurses of 79-A were no exception. It is one thing to look beautiful but quite another to be beautiful. And beautiful they were in every sense of the word.

Other families also were sitting quietly in the waiting room. They smiled knowingly as the Keatings entered. The Keatings returned their smiles and silently joined them. They attempted to look at magazines but found it hard to concentrate. Their minds jumped around with memories of the past, concerns of the present and the future, and thoughts of what might have been. Mike nervously roamed the halls for a while. Bored, he returned to leaf through a magazine, never seeing the images.

Suddenly, Dr. Hedlund appeared in the doorway. He looked serious, but his smile hinted that the surgery went okay. He came over and sat down next to the Keatings.

"Everything went well," he began. "We had to remove his entire left arm. We took it out of the shoulder so there will be no chance for a prosthesis. The leg was amputated at mid-calf but we might have to take more some time later. We need a minimum of about five centimeters below the knee for a prosthesis. We will reevaluate the situation after about a week. We have also cut slits along both sides of his leg." He demonstrated by running his index fingers along both the inside and outside of his leg. "This is necessary because of swelling and to relieve internal pressure."

He continued: "Another concern is the burn tissue itself. We will be grafting skin later. Yesterday's X-ray tests showed the bowels to be okay, but about 20 percent of the muscle tissue in the chest area was lost and had to be removed."

He paused allowing the couple to digest what they had just heard.

"The EKG was normal," he continued. "He remains on the kidney machine and respirator, but we hope to remove the respirator tonight or early tomorrow. In addition, we are going to attempt to bring him out of the medically induced coma in about 12 hours. His laboratory tests were as expected with no unexpected abnormalities, and his heart, blood pressure, and pulse are all normal. They were also strong and steady during the night."

He paused again and leaned back in his chair. "As to the future," he began, "the psychological shock of losing limbs can be devastating. We can discuss this again in a couple of days. There is a great mental plus if we can keep the leg amputation below the knee. This permits him to use his own knee when walking with a prosthesis. The next major concern is infection.

We will begin treating him with antibiotics in a few days. Infection is always a critical and major obstacle to survival for burn victims."

He again praised the emergency crew and the medical personnel for their outstanding initial treatment of John, emphasizing the fact that the first few hours are extremely critical for a burn victim. He reiterated John's youth was a major factor in his favor.

"His present condition is serious, and there could be kidney failure at any time," he warned.

"How about his heart?" asked Mike.

"The damage to the heart is still unknown. While the EKG is normal, we still must wait and see."

The Keatings thanked the doctor for his time and his frank medical explanation. As Dr. Hedlund was leaving, he turned and said, "Call Bosse tomorrow morning about 8:00 for an update."

* * *

You're tough and resilient, yet fun loving and easy-going (a rare combination). I know you'll pull through with flying colors.

—Bob Gabriel

* * *

The return trip to Stockholm was a little more upbeat due in part to the briefing Dr. Hedlund had given them and because they were to pick up Joanne at the Gushaws. John seemed to be holding his own considering his situation and, although there remained a lot of unanswered questions, there seemed to be hope. John had survived an eight-hour trip to the burn center and shown strong vital signs during the night as well as during the second surgery. These facts alone were encouraging. Mike and Judy looked forward to the next day when John hopefully would be conscious. It is one thing to see one's son in a coma, being kept alive by machines, and something else to see him conscious and responsive.

As Greg Gushaw welcomed them into his house, Joanne came running to greet them. She had been anxious and confused, but her mother sat down with her and explained everything that had happened, emphasizing the positive. She was very sad that her brother had lost his left arm and leg but was relieved that he was alive. She felt more secure now that she had seen her parents and would be going home with them to sleep in her own bed.

Carol had already departed for Finland on the evening ferryboat, and Greg was beginning to make a pizza for the girls.

"You'll stay for pizza, won't you?" he asked.

"I think we need to get home, we're dead tired. But thank you anyway," Mike replied.

"Joanne's been looking forward to pizza and I make it from scratch," he said with a smile, tossing the dough high in the air. "You know you're welcome, and it'll give you a chance to unwind a bit. Please reconsider."

Mike looked over at his wife and she smiled as if to say, *I feel relaxed in the love of this house.*

"Okay. I'll have a Bud!"

They left the Gushaws rejuvenated by the Gushaw milieu. They returned home and enjoyed a more relaxing sleep that night.

* * *

We're all fighting with you.

—*Jamie Sullivan*

* * *

"Hello, Bosse? This is Colonel Keating. How's John doing this morning?"

"He's doing fine. He's still in the process of waking up. The doctor removed the breathing tubes and he is breathing on his own now. Initially, it was very weak but when he was told to take a deep breath, he did. Not long ago he was asking about you. In response to his direct question if he had lost his arm and leg, I told him yes. His next question was if his parents knew, and I told him yes."

"When he is conscious again, you can tell him we'll be coming up to see him," Mike said.

"I'll tell him. He is lucid but tired. His spirits are good, but he seems very concerned about a Tim and Caroline."

"Those were two of the kids who were with him when the accident occurred."

"Oh! Okay. He's a fighter. He'll be remaining on the kidney machine until probably Monday, and we are feeding him directly into his small intestines via a tube."

"What's his medical classification?" asked Mike.

"Still listed as serious."

"Thanks, we'll see you all this afternoon."

Mike then called Erik Hammarskjold, a Swedish Coast Artillery major assigned to Fo/INT. He had been keeping Erik current on John's condition and Erik was passing the information to Admiral Algernon and the group still at Storlien. Mike was also keeping Chief Nowery informed since he was updating John's status and progress with the Defense Intelligence Agency, Headquarters USAF, and other interested parties both in Washington and in Europe.

* * *

We hope that his progress is miraculous—for all your sakes.

—Patti Curtis

* * *

When the Keatings arrived in Uppsala John was sleeping and, not wanting to disturb him, they adjourned to the waiting room. Several of the nurses came in and briefly expressed their sympathy and concern to Judy and Mike, encouraging them and wishing them strength. It was not that the nurses had time on their hands; they certainly did not. It was more of a genuine attachment they formed with all the patients and their families. These special people see many of their patients slip away, knowing there is little that the medical profession or anyone can do to save them. They have developed the ability to see through the horrible disfigurements and scars which burns leave on a victim and see the soul of a person who feels alone unto himself and who is as afraid of living as he is of dying. They give a lot more than just medical care to their patients, and when they lose one, they grieve as if they had lost someone very close.

One of the nurses popped her head through the door and said, "John's awake!"

Mike, Judy, and Joanne quickly followed the nurse down the hall towards John's room. Their anticipation grew with every step. Finally they would see and speak with their John. Each move seemed in slow motion as they hurriedly donned the sterile gowns, masks, and caps.

Finally dressed, they entered the room. John looked very weak and helpless tucked in between all the various pumping and beeping machines. He managed a faint smile.

"I'm sorry," he muttered weakly. "I'm so sorry."

Judy looked down into his teary eyes and said, "That's all right, John. Don't worry about it. Just get well!"

Tears welled up in Mike and Judy's eyes too—first tears of sorrow and then tears of happiness and joy. *He's going to make it!* they hoped. They recalled what Dr. Hedlund had told them earlier—that more burn victims die from infection than the actual trauma of the burn itself. They also recalled that he had said the emergency treatment John received had been excellent, that they were cultivating the bacteria from his wounds in order to determine the best combination of antibiotics, and that John had youth on his side. There was every reason to be optimistic.

Joanne was shocked to see all the life support machines and tubes running into her brother's body. She was unprepared for the encounter. Without a word, she left abruptly. She was simply overcome by the reality that John was seriously injured and was fighting for his life. She was experiencing the initial shock of the accident, not unlike Mike and Judy had at Storlien.

"Was it something I said?" John asked weakly.

"No. I think she was just scared. I'll talk to her," Judy answered.

John drifted off to sleep again as if he had been relieved of some heavy burden. He rested peacefully and looked contented.

"He needed to see us," Judy said as they left the room.

"Yes," Mike agreed.

"He needed to know we were okay with all that had happened."

"Yes," Mike repeated, reassuringly.

All of the Keatings had several more short visits that afternoon, and after each visit John seemed to look more relaxed and less worried.

* * *

You will be THE most important factor in his attitude. If he sees love and courage and confidence in him—in his being able to handle his adversity—then he'll be able to reflect it in showing you how he can grow and build from here and now.

—Barbara Leiser

* * *

Not long after returning home, the phone rang.

"Hi, Mike. This is Mary. We just got back from Storlien. How's John?"

Mary Thomson was the wife of the American Army Attaché, Colonel Bob Thomson. They were a very outgoing and fun-loving couple who were well received by the Swedes. An invitation to the Thomsons' home was a coveted one.

"John's doing okay," Mike answered. "We saw him this afternoon and he spoke to us. It's the first time he has been conscious. They have had him in a medical coma since the accident. Would you like to speak to Judy?"

"Yes."

"Hi, Mary. How was the trip?" said Judy.

"Enjoyed it immensely. Mike tells me John is doing okay."

"Yes. He'll be starting to fight infection in the next few days and that is a very critical time. But right now we are thankful that he is alive at all. The statistics on this type of accident are not at all encouraging. It is an exception to survive."

"Our prayers are with you all. You know that. Please let us take Joanne tomorrow and any other time you wish," Mary offered. "It must be hard on her and she's welcome here. Sitting around a hospital can be dreadful for her."

"I think she would enjoy spending tomorrow with you. Thank you for offering. We can drop her off on our way to Uppsala if that's okay."

"That will be great. Our prayers go out to you all. See you tomorrow."

Mike and Judy had delayed calling relatives and friends in the States because they wanted to have some type of definitive information to pass on. While John's life still hung in the balance, he had survived the first 48 hours and two operations. It was now time for them to call.

Mike called his brother Pat in Washington, D.C., to ask him to call Cannon Martin and St. Albans School. After a call to Mike's cousin, Pete Keating, in Wisconsin to ask him to relay the information to the Wisconsin relatives, Judy and Mike called Judy's brother Jack in New York to ask him to notify the New England relatives—Grandma Burgess, their mother, and their elder brother, Al. A call to Suzy

Hawley in Washington was next followed by a call to the Singers. The Singers were not at home, but Mike talked with Stephanie and gave her the news.

The calls were understandably difficult and emotional but at least they had some factual information to pass on, especially the news that John was alive. While everyone was shocked by the news, they were grateful and their genuine concern gave the Keatings strength. It had been reassuring and actually uplifting to know the concerns and prayers of those back in the States were with them. Two salient facts spurred them on: John was alive, and they had the support of those close to them.

* * *

I suppose tragedy has to be accepted and coped with but our hearts ache for all of you.

—Bernice Williams

* * *

It was Palm Sunday. Mike called Uppsala and spoke with Bosse. Bosse reported that John was very tired and had felt sick after drinking too much water. He also said they had changed the plasma going directly into John's leg and now hoped it would last the day.

After dropping Joanne off at the Thomsons, Mike and Judy headed for Uppsala. They were able to see John intermittently as he was still very tired and heavily medicated, drifting in and out of consciousness. Judy and Mike spent the majority of the time in the waiting room.

Sunday afternoons in a hospital are the same everywhere, and Sweden was no exception. Not much was going on. Most of the afternoon was spent talking to the nurses who admitted that it allowed them to practice their English, and they loved it.

As a *quid pro quo,* Judy seized the opportunity to practice her Swedish as well. They were impressed with her proficiency in their language, and they were quite interested in how she became so proficient. Judy then told them the story which Mike often used as a *tack for matten* at dinner parties. (*Tack for matten* translates to "thanks for the food" and is a short talk given by the senior or honored guest, thanking the host and hostess on behalf of all the guests. It normally includes a cute and humorous story.)

Mike often related that there were several valid reasons why his wife was more proficient in Swedish than he was. In the first place, he explained, women are more musically inclined than men and are better listeners. Therefore, women pick up the nuances, the rhythm, and the song of a language more easily. Like a child, they feel the language. In the second place, women are greater risk takers than men. In love, for example, women are the risk takers because they are the ones that bear the children. Men are often hooked into this "macho thing" and would never think of risking embarrassment by trying to use the language out in public. A woman, on the other hand, would not give it a second thought to walk into a grocery store and stumble through using a language they are attempting to learn. And finally, he concluded, "Judy is a whole lot smarter than I am."

The story, with its punch line of making himself the butt of the joke, always evoked laughter and applause.

Speaking Swedish to the nurses, Judy explained Mike's reasoning of why she was more proficient in Swedish than he, but apparently something was lost in the translation. She thought she had told them that women were like actresses trying out their skills and reading their audience to see how successfully they communicated. Several months later she learned to her surprise that the word around the hospital was that "the American's" mother was an actress!

*   *   *

John is a super person, full of spirit, determination, and a strong ability to cope. With these qualities, he will handle himself, overcoming any adversity that tries to stand in his way.

—Mary Cronin

* * *

On the way home and before stopping by the Thomsons to pick up Joanne, Mike and Judy swung by the home of Calle and Margaretta Algernon in Taby, a suburb of Stockholm. The Admiral and his wife had just returned from Storlien the previous afternoon.

The Keatings had first met the Admiral and his wife in Washington at the home of Titti and Lennart Forsman, the Swedish Defense Attaché in Washington. At that time the Admiral was the Director of Intelligence for the Defense Staff and a person with whom Mike would work rather closely. The Admiral subsequently became the Director of the Defense International Office and their close contact continued. The 1981 Winter Trip was the last official function of the Algernons in his position as Director of Fo/INT. He was moving over to become Director of Sweden's Foreign Military Assistance Office. The Algernon family was very close, and the Admiral included the foreign military attachés and their families in many of the official attaché functions. He once remarked to Judy that her John reminded them of their eldest son, Johan.

Mike and Judy wanted to stop by for a brief minute to personally update them on John's condition and to assure them that they were coping. When the Admiral opened the door, he called to his wife, "Margaretta, it's Mike and Judy." The two couples stood in the entryway; not a word was spoken. They simply hugged each other and wept.

* * *

There is in Washington, and colleges all over, a great network of people trying somehow to get their love to John over thousands of miles.

—Maxine Singer

* * *

Knowing how important it was for John to see Caroline and Tim, and how much they needed to see him, Judy called them Sunday night to ask if they would like to accompany her and Colonel Keating to Uppsala Monday afternoon to visit John.

"Colonel Keating is going into the Embassy Monday morning, and we are going to see John in the afternoon. Would you two like to join us?" she asked.

"We sure would," Caroline replied.

"John has been asking about you for the last couple of days, and I think it would do him a world of good to see you two before you return to England."

"Oh! Great! Thank you for thinking of us. We can hardly wait."

"John's very weak and heavily medicated so he drifts off every once in a while. We only spend about 10 to 15 minutes with him at a time. He'll be quite pleased to see you. See you tomorrow then."

When Mike arrived at the office Monday morning he was swamped by well-wishers, and he found it difficult to hold back the tears since many of the visitors were very emotional. He had been in constant contact with Chief Nowery, and the Chief had kept the Embassy updated. After meeting with the DAO personnel, Mike dropped by the Chargé d'Affaires' office to personally brief him on John's progress. He then returned to his office where he began returning calls from many Swedish friends and attaché associates who had called to offer their best wishes. One of the calls was to Fo/INT.

"Hello, Major Hall speaking."

"Ove, this is Mike Keating. How are you doing?"

"I'm good, sir. How are you and Mrs. Keating? And John?"

"We're doing all right. John is slowly making progress, and we are now preparing to ride out the onslaught of infection. The doctors tell us this is the most critical time," Mike said.

"I called really to thank you for your and Ingemar's Herculean efforts on our behalf," he continued. "The arrangements you all made—the taxi, the travel, the staying with us the entire time, the support, and the logistics of getting Judy and Joanne and our stuff back to Stockholm, all were fantastic. We cannot even begin to thank you enough for all your effort and kindness. The Keating family will always be indebted to you and, in fact, to all of Fo/INT for their support in this very trying time for us."

"I was glad I could help and am honored that your call for help was to me," Ove replied.

"Thank you, Ove."

"I would very much like to visit John sometime if it could be arranged. When can he have visitors?" Ove asked.

"That can be arranged," Mike replied. "We are taking Caroline and Tim up there this afternoon as John has been asking about them. Both Judy and I feel that while the visits must be necessarily short because he tires quickly, it gives him reassurance to see those who were with him in Storlien. It is also reassuring for them to see John. We would be pleased if you could visit him also. He is aware of the role you played, and I know he would like personally to thank you. You are welcome at any time. You can come up this afternoon if you wish."

"That would be fantastic. I'll be there. Thank you so much."

* * *

You are all too strong and too tough not to pick up the pieces and continue.

—Suki Reynolds

* * *

While the visitors had to take turns visiting John because of all the medical paraphernalia in his room, John was very pleased to see Caroline and Tim again and to learn they were handling the tragedy well. Likewise, the two British youngsters were delighted to see John. It provided a closure for them, a kind of relief so that they could return to school in England the following week with the knowledge that they had seen John alive and had spoken to him.

While John did not really know Ove Hall, he recognized him and thanked him for all his and Ingemar's help. John also was very grateful that he cared enough to follow up with a visit to see him. The visits were a great boost for everyone, John in particular.

While the visits were taking place, the Keatings met with Dr. Hedlund and Dr. Skogs, the orthopedic surgeon. The doctors informed them that they would have to remove more of John's leg, possibly on Thursday, explaining that dead tissue was causing further damage to the healthy tissue.

"We'll be starting an antibiotic protocol this week," Dr. Hedlund said. "We are also feeding him through a tube in his nose rather than directly into his small intestines."

Dr. Skogs nodded as Hedlund continued, "The kidneys look good but the heart is still a question mark since the EKGs vary. There could be some minor damage but we'll just have to wait and see. We'll be doing skin grafting later also."

* * *

> *...recognize that your recovery—and you will recover!!—must come from your own (and your family's) strength and determination.*
>
> *—Pete Keating*

* * *

Judy continued to make the hour drive daily to Uppsala to visit John while Mike returned to work. Initially, he took one or two afternoons off each week to visit John, and of course they both would visit him on weekends and on days of surgery. They attempted to maintain as much of a normal routine as they could. They resumed their social functions in order to keep their friends and acquaintances apprised of John's status and to receive their greetings and good wishes to pass on to John. It was not an easy task for the Keatings, but the message they were sending to John was that they were coping and he should not worry about them.

Many of John's friends wanted to visit him, but the Keatings recognized that his visitors had to be restricted. He would tire easily and would expend a lot of energy trying to convince them that he was okay. So his parents began controlling John's visitors. They explained to John that it was their job to cheer people up and his job to get well.

On Tuesday, April 14th, Bo Rybeck, the Swedish Surgeon General, called Mike from his office in Karlstad to offer encouragement and any assistance he could. He had been in contact with the Hospital in Uppsala and was very encouraged by the reports he was receiving. He also offered that he personally knew Dr. Pruitt, the Chief of the Burn Center at Brooke Army Hospital, and that the Swedish protocol in the treatment of burns was the same as that at Brooke. He said he would forward some literature on rehabilitation.

John was gaining strength day by day, and it was evident. He had more energy and could withstand visits for longer periods. During one of his mother's visits, he related what he remembered of when he first arrived in the Burn Unit. Judy was amazed that he had any memory of his arrival because he had been unconscious at the time.

"I remember I was entering the double doors and all these medical people in scrubs were rushing around and taking care of me," John said. "I was aware of other spirits or souls around but nobody was paying attention to any of them. I didn't understand why the staff didn't help them also. The medical people were attending only to me.

"At that moment, I realized I was alive, and they were trying to save me but that the others had been lost. They were dead," he concluded.

On a later occasion he related, "I was aware of floating, the sensation of floating. I was bathed in a warm light, secure and peaceful. I felt reassured, loved, supported, and tremendous outside strength. I was aware of a voice, a familiar voice calling my name, but I just can't remember whose voice it was. I knew I was going to be okay even though I was hearing myself saying, *I'm not going to make it.*"

Judy was deeply touched by this revelation, and it gave her reassurance. Her prayers had been for strength for John and for his survival. Following the amputations, as she worried about what kind of life was ahead for him, she released her own desires—"Thy will be done." She accepted the fact that the battle was John's, and the matter was out of her hands. His survival was in the hands of God.

John also spoke of a recurring nightmare he was having. He said he was constantly searching for his cowboy hat that he had been wearing at the time of the accident. In his dream, the hat was the key to his survival. He would die if he could not find it.

Tim and Caroline, as well as Ove Hall, were aware that the hat was missing and had returned to the scene of the accident to look for it. They walked along the tracks searching for the hat the following day. In addition, they had asked around but to no avail. No one had seen it. The hat had disappeared.

The hat had been a graduation gift from Bitsy Cronin, John's high school girl friend, and was obviously very meaningful to him. The hat's importance to John's recovery was passed on by Mike to friends in Washington. Finally, here was something tangible his friends back home could do to reach out to John. A plan began to form.

John was progressing, as evidenced by his concern about his appearance. When he had arrived at the hospital, the medical personnel had to shave the front part of his head along the hairline in order to treat a wound he had received during his fall. Not liking this bald spot, John asked his parents to bring him his fraternity baseball cap. John had pledged Tau Kappa Epsilon (TKE), and the cap had the two-inch letters boldly embossed across the front.

The University Hospital in Uppsala was a teaching hospital and, as such, when the doctors made their rounds they were followed by a group of interns and residents. The entourage of doctors reminded John of a gaggle of geese as they entered his room and encircled his bed.

The day after his mother brought him the cap, Dr. Hedlund came into John's room with the gaggle tagging along. After discussing the case, he turned to John and asked, "What does TKE stand for?"

"TEN THOUSAND KILOVOLTS OF ELECTRICITY!" John replied.

Hedlund laughed, and as he left the room he could be heard still chuckling to himself as he shook his head back and forth. With the bevy of doctors who had witnessed this exchange, it did not take long for that story to get around the hospital. The legend of "the American" was forming.

On Thursday, John developed a fever. The infections had begun and the doctors immediately adjusted his antibiotic therapy. John did not feel well and was distressed fearing something was going wrong. His parents explained that everyone had been anticipating this situation and the doctors were more than able to deal with it. Even with the reassurance of his parents, he still worried—but not as much as they did.

* * *

You have my tears and my smiles and my prayers. Take as much as you need, I have an endless supply. Don't ever hesitate to ask, please.

—Drew Fleishmann

* * *

Meanwhile back in the United States, the logistics of procuring a new cowboy hat and expeditiously getting it to Ward 79-A in Uppsala, Sweden, took on a rather high priority among some government agencies and friends of John. Bitsy's mother, Mary Cronin, contacted her daughter at the University of Alabama in Tuscaloosa for a description of the hat. She also contacted Dave Singer, who was going to be home from Yale over the Passover weekend, to come by the house to give his approval to the one she had picked out at Count's Western. She had called Suzy Hawley as well and discussed the transportation options. Mike had been in contact with Dick McHargue, the Defense Intelligence Agency's Desk Officer for the Eastern Bloc and Neutral Countries in Europe. Dick was a can-do type of individual, the "go-to guy" when the game is on the line. Mike asked him to contact Suzy Hawley and see if a rendezvous could be arranged for the hat to be passed to him so that he could get it in the diplomatic pouch.

"Consider it done," Dick said.

* * *

John, we are thinking of you with constant love and faith in your resourcefulness and strength. Wish we were closer.

—Suzy Hawley

* * *

The following Saturday, John complained that he did not feel well and had chills just after he was given his antibiotic medications. His mother noticed a skin rash beginning to show, swelling in his face, and welts forming on his foot.

He's having a reaction to the medication, she thought. She summoned one of the nurses.

The nurse came in, examined him, and said, "He's feverish. Looks like it might be a reaction to the antibiotics. I'll call the doctor."

She left immediately and called for another nurse to monitor John while she called the bacteriologist. The doctor was working in his garden when the call came. He dropped everything and left for the hospital, arriving in John's room in about 20 minutes. Fortunately John's reaction had not progressed to a state of anaphylaxis. The doctor examined him thoroughly and gave orders to discontinue the treatment until they could determine what was causing the reaction. The culprit was found to be Cephalosporins, which was eliminated from the treatment. John responded, and within a few days had beaten the infection.

* * *

> *Praise God he is alive and also that you do have such a great support from all of those close who care.*
>
> —*Barbara Burman*

* * *

When the Keatings returned home from Uppsala, they had no sooner entered their house than the front doorbell rang. It was their neighbors, Rolf and Anna Lena Berg. Rolf was an inventor and businessman, well known in Sweden for inventing the candle-like-flickering electric light bulb, the plastic credit card for medical identification, and an extrusion technique in the manufacture of seamless aluminum cans. They were a delightful couple and great neighbors. They had a picnic basket, sent out from Ostermalm, chock full of shrimp, bread, salad, wine, everything for a picnic.

"We've brought a picnic for you," Rolf announced. "We want you to relax and enjoy the remainder of the day."

It was quite a shock because the Swedes in general are not spontaneous. This is something they would not normally do, but Rolf was not your typical Swede. While he was very formal, polite, and proper, he enjoyed being different, unique, and spontaneous. The two couples laid out the tablecloth and sat down to a delightful evening of much needed relaxation. The timing could not have been better—it was just the kind of evening the Keatings needed to recharge their batteries.

* * *

The message of Easter is that hope is born out of despair and the darkness.

—The Reverend Christopher Frey

* * *

Sunday was Easter and the Easter Bunny had left a card written in a handwriting that looked suspiciously like Joanne's. The card read:

Dear Mom & Dad,
I hope you have a very nice Easter and
many more in the following years to come.
Say hi to John and Joanne.
Love,
The Easter Bunny

The Keatings had invited the Landergrens and Barcilons, along with their families, for an Easter Brunch. Since the invitations had gone out a week or so before the Winter Trip, both Christina Landergren and Jacquie Barcilon called politely inquiring as to whether the lunch was going to be cancelled. Judy explained that John was making progress and the knowledge that his parents were maintaining "business as usual" would be reassuring to him. It would signal to him that they believed he was progressing and on his way to recovery. The brunch would go on as scheduled.

General Nils Landergren had been the Commander of the Stockholm Garrison and had just recently replaced Admiral Algernon as the Director of Fo/INT. He was a tall, thin, stately man, and his charming wife Christina had the energy of a teenager. The Landergrens had entertained the Keating family, along with their houseguest, Dave Singer, during the Christmas vacation in 1979. At the time, both John and Dave were quite smitten with the Landergrens' lovely daughter Cecilia.

Group Captain Robert Barcilon was the British Defense and Air Attaché, Mike's counterpart in the British Embassy. Both he and his lovely wife Jacquie were very close to the Keatings and were of great comfort to them during this entire ordeal. They also had suffered a tragedy previously when the fiancé of their eldest daughter, Nichola, had been killed in a skydiving accident.

The brunch was relaxing and very enjoyable. It was a family affair which included the Landergrens' three children: Cecilia, Fredrik, and Catharina; Catharina's husband Johan and their baby daughter Michaela. The Barcilons' youngest daughter Rae-Louise and her friend from England, Emma Knight, joined in making it a family affair—a reminder of the innate strength to be found within the family. After the guests departed, Mike, Judy, and Joanne headed for Uppsala to visit John.

John had asked one of the nurses to pick up an Easter card for him to give his parents. He looked forward with anticipation to surprising them. He was quite pleased with himself and when they arrived that afternoon, he could hardly contain himself. His Mom opened the card and read:

Dear Mom and Dad,
Thank you all so very much.
I love you with all my heart.
Happy Easter.
John

It was a very special and emotional moment for all of them. John had indeed surprised his parents with his thoughtfulness and consideration in view of everything he had endured the past week and a half.

After his parents departed to return to Stockholm, John propped himself up with a pillow and wrote:

John Keating
Akademiska Sjukhuset
Uppsala, Sweden

April 19, 1981

Dearest Suzy (and Mark, Pete, Dave),

First of all, let me thank you for your telegram and your efforts to continue to convey information through the Singers. Thank you very much. It really did feel warm and frighteningly pleasing to hear you all were so concerned. Second, let me say I'm sorry about the penmanship here but I'm just only now starting to write again and I'm finding it very difficult.

As you know the accident was quite a terrible thing, but now I'm already standing (with support) and can move from bed to chair by myself.

I'm still having a lot of pain all the time and the nightmares are by far the worst and most painful. I'm having what is called phantom pains in my left arm (hand in particular) and in my left foot.

I'm recovering rapidly and they (the doctors) plan on more surgery and skin grafting on my left leg this week. They say it should help to ease the pain and also make it look better.

I worry about Mom and Dad. I think I'm doing fine and improving at an incredible rate, but Mom and Dad must face the world each day and people must be constantly questioning them and I'm sure they have a lot on their minds. But I love them. I get strength from them, and I love you and can feel the same strength from you.

Love and kisses,
John

P.S. **Pete:** *You know every day I see about 20-25 different nurses. Each day!!! Man! All are fantastic, not a rotten apple in the bunch. And all from 20-34, most 20-24. Come see!*

* * *

> *Through one of Maxine's colleagues at NIH—who has a friend at Uppsala Hospital—we got a very upbeat report indicating John is out of danger...That's encouraging and hopeful. Also, the report was that the doctor in charge of John's case is one of the world's best and that the Burn Unit is outstanding.*
>
> *—Dan Singer*

* * *

Stephanie Singer
Washington, D.C.

April 11, 1981

Dear Johnny,

Smile! Because wherever you go and whatever happens, there are a lot of people back here in D.C. who think about you often.

Your father called this afternoon to tell Dave of your accident. I was the only one home. I drove down to the dorms to tell Ernie and I stood around talking to him and some other guys but we really didn't talk, we just stood there until someone said, "Damn, why do things always happen to the best guys?"

I just wanted to write and tell you that I care and I'm thinking of you and don't let appearances kid you—you're still a Freebird.

Love,
Stephanie

* * *

TDMT NEW HAVEN CT 34/32 12 0710P EST
JOHN KEATING CARE COLONEL MICHAEL KEATING
AMERICAN EMBASSY S11527 STOCKHOLM

WE ALL LOVE YOU AND ARE THINKING ABOUT YOU AND JOANNE MOM AND DAD.

STARSKY WIGGY MIKE CARL CHRIS AND JUSTIN

* * *

National Cathedral School for Girls
Washington, D.C.

April 12, 1981

Dear John!

We just wanted to let you know that we are all thinking of you and praying for you—

Feel

Better

Soon !!!

Love,
The Class of '81 NCS

*　　*　　*

Maxine Singer
Washington, D.C.

April 12, 1981

Dear John,

We're all thinking about you. If thinking and loving help, you can't help improving every day! Remember we're all counting on you and your great spirit to see mending well and soon.

Love,
Maxine & Dan Singer

* * *

Maxine Singer
Washington, D.C.

April 12, 1981

Dear Judy and Mike,

There is here in Washington, and at colleges all over, a great network of people trying somehow to get their love to John over thousands of miles. That marvelous group of young men from St. Albans, class of 1980, are sorely frustrated by not being able to come immediately to be with all of you. They really are unique in the way they care for each other.

Dan and I, too, want you both to know how much our thoughts are with you.

Yours,
Maxine Singer

* * *

TDMT BOXFORD MA 32/31 13 0841A EST VIA RCA
JOHN KEATING
AMERICAN EMBASSY STRANDVAGEN 101 S115 27 STOCKHOLM

JOHN AND FAMILY

YOUR EXTENDED FAMILY SENDS WELL WISHES. YOU ARE ALL IN OUR THOUGHTS AND PRAYERS.

LOVE

AUNT CAROLYN UNCLE AL

* * *

TF BETHESDA MARYLAND 32 15 430 P
JOHN KEATING C/O COL KEATING
AMERICAN EMBASSY STOCKHOLM

LOVE, THOUGHTS AND PRAYERS FOR OUR JOHN. YOU WILL ALWAYS HAVE A SPECIAL PLACE IN OUR HEARTS.

MARY AND DON CRONIN AND LIZZIE

* * *

TDMT ALEXANDRIA VA 40/37 15 0936P EST
KEATINGS AMERICAN EMBASSY STOCKHOLM

JOHN WE ARE THINKING OF YOU WITH CONSTANT LOVE AND FAITH IN YOUR RESOURCEFULNESS AND STRENGTH. WISH WE WERE CLOSER.

MRS ROBINSON, HAWLEYS AND WISES

* * *

James P. Keating
Neenah, Wisconsin

April 13, 1981

Dear John,

Your Dad phoned last Saturday to tell us about your accident, both the bad news that you've suffered burns and loss of limbs, and the ***good*** *news that you're alive!!!*

The ***best*** *news we could have heard is that you survived an experience that would have killed a lesser man, and that you are lucid, responding to treatment with a prognosis of good recovery.*

This is important as hell, John, because we all learn to adjust to what ***other*** *people call "handicaps". Virtually* ***any physical*** *shortcoming can be adjusted to and eventually neutralized.*

You'll encounter well-meaning people who will try to smother you with sympathy and attempt to do everything for you. Be kind, but recognize that your recovery—and you ***will*** *recover!!!—must come from your own (and your family's) strength and determination.*

Once you're into the physical therapy part of all of this, and they fit you with some of the damnedest prosthetic contraptions you've ever seen, you'll have some tangible goals to shoot for.

Sometimes the ways of life on this "poor old earth" work in strange ways. Some of us are given mountains to climb—damn ***big*** *mountains—but climb them we will.*

Focus on the ***future****, John; your education, career, friends, family.* ***These*** *are the important things, along with your faith and the guts I know you have.*

Keep us posted on your progress. Our prayers for your recovery go with you.

Love,
Aunt Sally & Uncle Pete

*　　　*　　　*

Bernice Williams
Neenah, Wisconsin

April 13, 1981

Dear Judy and Mike,

Pete called us Saturday p.m. What a shock! I really don't know what to say. Pete said not to call you until next week, or later. You know that our thoughts are with you, and we wish we could comfort you and help you through this. My heart aches for Joanne too—how is she?

The fact that John is alive means everything, I know—and wonderful recoveries are made. You are both very strong people and John is a boy with lots of grit and stamina—so now—we hope and pray.

We'll keep in touch.

Our love to all of you,
Bernice

*　　　*　　　*

Dale Banfield
Holten-Arms School
Bethesda, Maryland

April 14, 1981

Dear John,

Hey! I bet you never expected to hear from me! When I heard what had happened to you—I prayed to God that you'd be all right and thanked Him that you were still alive. Well cutie, my prayers were answered! I hear you're doin' well and let me tell you—I'm so happy!

I know I don't know you very well but ever since I visited you in the hospital last year—you've been nice to me and I think you're pretty damn special!

One thing I admire so much about you is your zest for life! I love it! I look up to people like you 'cause that's what I want to be like! I also know that you won't let what happened to you interfere with the rest of your life—that's why I think you're so great! YOU AMAZE ME BOY!!!

I know I haven't done much but I hope I've cheered you up! Believe me, everything I've said has come straight from my heart! I meant every word of this!

Please take care and God bless you, John.

All my love,
Dale

P.S. I remember when you kissed my hand in the hospital! I haven't washed it since then!! (No! I'm not that dizzy!) REMEMBER:

Whenever you want me, I'll be there.
Whenever you need me, I'll be there.

Whenever you want me, I'll be there.
I'll be around.

* * *

Mrs. Walter Burgess
Union, Maine

April 14, 1981

My Dear Grand Children:

A few lines to let you know I am stunned by the terrible tragedy that has happened to John. I just can't realize it; I can hardly even believe it. Why? Why? Why?

Why are you afflicted with these ills and injuries to cause such heartaches? Words are so inadequate at times like this, what message may I send to let you know how sorry I am for all of you. I hope Sadie will write you. We all in the USA will be so anxious to hear more details on the accident and how John is getting along. If we could only help, do let us know if there is anything we can do. What would John like?

I do hope he will not suffer, be kept under opiates—I just can't realize it and what it will do to his life. We can be thankful it was no worse—certainly bad enough. Words can't express how sorry I am and I know all of your folks in the USA are too.

I'll put in a check for a bit, you will know what to get John. Tell him we are thinking of him many times a day and hoping in time things will get better. We think of Joanne and hope this does not upset her also.

This isn't much of a note but to let you know we are thinking of you all and hoping for better news before long. What do you have—about 15 months more in Sweden? Sorry, sorry for all this trouble.

Take care the best you can. Thinking of you all with much love,
Grandma Burgess

* * *

Drew Fleischmann
Bethesda, Maryland

April 14, 1981

Dear John,

I've never been particularly good with words, and I can't pretend that I am now—but I do want you to know that I care. I care very much, so does everybody. The sympathy you have here is overwhelming. Whether you realize it or not, you have a lot of friends and a lot of support.

I know I'm not saying anything original. What I would like to say, I can't; there aren't the words to replace sitting by a bed or holding a hand. At any rate, if there are, I'm not aware of them.

You have my tears and my smiles and my prayers. Take as much as you need, I have an endless supply. Don't ever hesitate to ask, please. I'm not real outspoken—like I said, I'm afraid of words—but just because I don't always say them doesn't mean the thoughts aren't there.

I know you can't possibly answer all the letters you receive. Don't even try. Just remember that I am here for you now and later. We all are.

Best wishes,
Druenette

* * *

Suzy Hawley
Alexandria, Virginia

April 17, 1981

Dearest Keatings,

My goodness, how well loved you are! Just got a call from Mary Cronin who is trying to figure out the best and fastest way to get the new cowboy hat to John. She was full of all sorts of love and good things to say about John—how polite he is, etc.! (Fooled her, didn't he!!) I guess the Singers gave her my number. Singers are wonderful!! Talked to Pat several times. He's going to call you today. Called Sandra and Jack after I talked with you. She's lovely…didn't talk with Jack. Glad I got to meet her. Promised to send her the Swedish tray.

Am contemplating coming to see you about the 2nd or 3rd week in July. Dave gets home the 1st of July. Would it be helpful or a hindrance? The last thing I want is to be in the way—but thought maybe it would be good to have a different face around to lend a hand and lots of love. Let me know and I'll start to make plans.

Am about on my way to Lexington. Have so much more to clean out. Pa's champing at the bit because he is about to remarry and is trying to get everything set. Had the house repainted inside last week and Ann's furniture is about to arrive. He brought her here for a weekend—and I had to ask that they not sleep together in the same room with teen-age boys here. For some reason that statement seemed crazy!! Anyway, they're absolutely devoted to each other—and roaring around the country—and the world! She is delightful—62, very attractive and a super sense of humor. Wish Mum had had the same opportunity.

Write when you can. Thinking of you all constantly.

Love,
Suzy

* * *

Mary Cronin
Bethesda, Maryland

April 18, 1981

Dear Col. and Mrs. Keating,

There are times when words cannot adequately describe one's feelings and thoughts. What we, Don, Bitsy and I, feel for John and for you are love and support. John is a super person, full of spirit, determination, and a strong ability to cope. With these qualities he will handle himself, overcoming any adversity that tries to stand in his way.

Bitsy said to me over the phone that the Keatings are so mentally and physically strong, as well as supportive—qualities everyone desires to possess—and she hoped she married someone of such great strength and character. John is lucky to have parents like you. He has inherited these innate, superior properties that will encourage him to succeed.

I will be sending John's hat in the next few days. Dave Singer came by this morning to approve it, as I wanted to replace his as closely as possible. Should it be a bit snug, it can be stretched or padded if too large. I hope you will let me know if there is something more we can do for John or for you.

Love to you both and Joanne. Our prayers are with you all.

Fondly,
Mary Cronin

*　　*　　*

John C. Davis
St. Albans School
Washington, D.C.

April 19, 1981

Dear John,

You must forgive me for typing my letter since I am not sure that emotion would have permitted me to write it in longhand.

You are so fortunate to have the parents you have, who have given you a great deal of strength and character, and I am sure it will gradually become more apparent to you what you have received from them.

Ultimately, I guess, the bottom line will be yourself, and I am also confident—as you recall I was in the past two years at St. Albans—that you will emerge from this much stronger than you were when you left St. Albans.

I have become increasingly aware, as I have been watching my 92-year-old mother gradually disintegrate into senility, that one should be always grateful for the situation as it now is, regardless of what the disadvantages are and seem to be, because there are worse things. I don't have to tell you this, I know, but a reminder may be helpful. I once went up on a mountain outside of Cortona, Italy, with a St. Albans graduate whom I was traveling with. The night was very dark, and the lights of the Tuscan plain stretched out to the horizon, and I suddenly became conscious of the beauty of that particular moment. And then I realized that every moment of life has to be realized as beautiful, without regret for the past or worry of the future, and that the NOW is the chief moment to be enjoyed.

It is hard perhaps for you to see this, or if you have, I just wanted to reinforce what is perhaps in your own mind. But just remember that you are 19 or 20, you are attractive and that people will love you not for what you have lost but for what you have, and that you have so much to look forward to in your future. You also have the potential to develop yourself as a beautiful person inside, and that—believe it or not—is what is now given to you.

Please keep this note for yourself. I will write your parents. Just give them my affection, and keep a little or even a lot for yourself. You are so fortunate in so many ways.

As ever,
John Davis

P.S. I shall be at STA over the summer, and whatever I can do for you, please let me know. I'd have time to write if you like, and I hope to see you when you get back if you let me know when. Should your therapy require your presence in Washington, and the educational side of things is feasible again, let me know right away so I can start things moving with a possible transcript application to one of the local universities. There is some merit in going to one of them, should that be in your plans. Think about it.

John

* * *

CHAPTER THREE

Ward 79-A
(April 20–May 8, 1981)

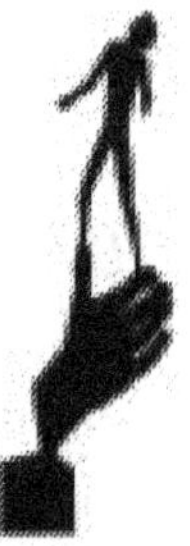

*　　　　*　　　　*

...when word of your accident spread at school, several people said to me that there was no one in the Class of '80 who would be stronger or better able to bounce back from such an ordeal than John Keating.

—Mark Mullin

*　　　　*　　　　*

The role the nurses played in John's recovery was certainly more than just their medical expertise. They soon found "the American" to be an enjoyable and entertaining challenge, and they respected his zest for life and his sense of humor. Several commented to his parents that he epitomized the Spirit of America with all its hopes, its dreams, and its optimistic promises for the future. As far as the nurses of 79-A were concerned, there was never any doubt that "the American" was going to make it.

The Swedes have always felt rather close to the Americans. After all, almost everyone in Sweden had some distant relative who had immigrated to the United States. During the early twentieth century, 20 percent of the population of Sweden emigrated seeking the opportunities and promises the new country had to offer. It was that kindred spirit the nurses shared with John. They understandably felt possessive of all their patients because they daily witnessed and affected the delicate life-and-death balance, which their wards had to negotiate. In addition, John was a contemporary, a young adult not unlike them, with all the hopes and dreams of the future.

John had his own descriptive method of identifying the nurses. He did not use their names when talking to his parents and friends—he preferred to refer to them by how they "appeared" to him. There was the Night Nurse, Lilla Mor, Miss Sweden, Bedroom Eyes, Tinker Bell, and the Goalie.

The Night Nurse was a shift supervisor. She was older than the other nurses, probably in her thirties. She lived with her husband on a farm outside Uppsala. Just after John had the feeding tubes removed and had begun to take liquids by mouth, the Night Nurse brought him a special Swedish dessert made from the first milk of a cow that has just given birth. It is a special, old-world elixir, loaded with vitamins and believed to have healing powers far beyond anything modern medicine can provide. Mike and Judy were very touched by her concern and thoughtful gesture.

Lilla Mor is a Swedish term meaning "Little Mother," and this nurse was certainly that. She like the others was a beautiful, caring individual who had all the motherly attributes. She was constantly checking on John—"Are you all right?" asking questions—"Is there anything I can get you? Are you comfortable?" and giving instructions—"John, you need to eat more in order to get stronger."

Miss Sweden, as the name implies, was gorgeous, a jewel among jewels. While any of the nurses could hold their own in any beauty contest, Miss Sweden, at five foot-eleven, towered above them and had been awarded the title by John. She was a good listener and spent time one-on-one with John, permitting him to express his feelings about the loss of his arm and leg. This time together enabled John to examine his situation and feelings without all the emotions involved in discussing the subject with his parents. It permitted him to accept his misfortune and get on with his recovery and his life. One day towards the end of his stay on the fifth floor, Miss Sweden proudly announced to John's parents that she had "bath-ed" John all by herself. The Keatings were initially slightly taken aback, wondering if, with her beauty and sex appeal, this was a good thing; but then they chuckled as she glowed with pride at her accomplishment. Normally, it took two or three nurses to bathe a burn patient because of all the mechanical lifts involved. Miss Sweden, with the help and assistance of her patient, had accomplished the task by herself.

Sally and Mike Hare, the British Naval Attaché, and their children had been on the trip to Storlien and after returning to Stockholm, the children had collected an assortment of items for John's amusement. One of the items was a small white rubber mouse. One morning, Bedroom Eyes, with her seductively innocent, doe-like eyes, had just begun to change John's dressings when John complained that something felt funny under the bandage on his leg. As Bedroom Eyes was carefully unwrapping the bandage, John flipped out the little white mouse with his finger. The nurse screamed and fell back against the wall, arms raised above her head. She was frozen there with a look of stark terror. Just then the parade of doctors entered to find the frightened nurse backed against the wall and "the American" lying in his bed laughing. After an explanation of what had just happened, Dr. Hedlund said, "That's okay, John. You're allowed to do that."

Bedroom Eyes had recovered sufficiently by this time and regained her composure enough to enjoy the moment. She smiled at John and sternly said, "John, I don't know what we're going to do with you."

As the doctors were leaving, Dr. Hedlund turned to John and asked, "How are the nurses treating you?"

"They're taking good care of me," John replied. He paused, smiled, glanced at Bedroom Eyes and added, "So far!"

The Goalie was an athletic, auburn-haired beauty. She played ice hockey during the winter and was the goalie on a local soccer team in the spring and summer. She, like the rest of the nurses, took an interest in John and even observed a couple of his operations after he had been transferred from the burn unit to the surgical ward. One day when John was in recovery, she came into the waiting room and announced, "John can ride a bike!"

She went on to explain to Judy and Mike that she had ridden her bike to work that day using only one leg and one arm. Therefore, she concluded that John could ride a bike.

"I tried it and he can," she proclaimed.

When Judy related this revelation to John later in the day, his comment was, "Why in the world would I want to ride a bike?"

* * *

I just wanted to write and tell you that I care and I'm thinking of you and don't let appearances kid you—you're still a Freebird.
—Stephanie Singer

* * *

In Washington, Suzy Hawley and Mary Cronin had decided to meet for lunch in Georgetown. They had been talking on the phone almost daily since the news of the accident and wanted a chance to meet face to face. In addition, Mary wanted to show Suzy the cowboy hat before her rendezvous with Dick McHargue later that day.

Because of the traffic and parking problems in Washington in general and Rosslyn in particular, Dick told Suzy he would meet Mary on Lynn Street between 19th Street and Wilson Boulevard. Mary was to pull her car over into the bus/taxi lane and up to the curb in the middle of the block at the appointed time. Dick would pick up the package through the passenger-side window, and Mary could be on her way without a hassle. Unfortunately, Mary was not that familiar with Rosslyn, so after lunch Suzy had Mary follow her to the drop point.

They laughed during lunch about this scenario of dropping off an unmarked box containing a cowboy hat to a member of the Defense Intelligence Agency whom neither had ever seen and only one had spoken to in a city known for its intrigue and mystery. Fortunately, the drop went off as planned, and as Suzy glanced in her rear view mirror, she chuckled as this man in a trench coat reached into Mary's open car window and retrieved the package. The hat was on its way.

* * *

Nobody says you must laugh, but a sense of humor can help you overlook the unattractive, tolerate the unpleasant, and smile through the unbearable.

—Unknown, sent by Justin Walker

* * *

Surgery had been scheduled for Wednesday, the 22nd, but was postponed since John was still taking antibiotics. The doctors rescheduled it for Monday, the 27th.

Tinker Bell and the Goalie greeted John as they entered his room. They placed his records on his stomach and began moving him and his bed down to the operating room. They were upbeat and cheerful. When they arrived at the surgical suite, they positioned John in a small staging area, wished him luck, and departed.

John lay there for a while but soon became curious and decided to look at his records. He opened them up and discovered several sheets of photographs taken upon his arrival at the burn unit. The pictures were graphic, and John suddenly realized the extent to which he had been injured. He closed the records placing them back on his stomach. He felt blessed that he had survived.

A short time later, two surgical nurses moved John into the operating room. He recognized Drs. Skogs and Hedlund, who began explaining to John what they were planning to do. John listened to the doctor intently, and when he had finished, announced, "I looked at the pictures in my records."

A sudden look of concern fell across Dr. Hedlund's face. He looked around the room as if to determine who had been responsible for such a breech of protocol. The surgical team did not miss his "how-did-this-happen" look, and the atmosphere became tense.

"The pictures were appalling," John proclaimed.

"I know," replied Dr. Hedlund. "I'm sorry. You should not have been allowed to see them."

"There isn't a single one of me smiling," John complained.

The tension immediately lifted as a titter ran through the operating room. "The American" and the surgical team were now ready to proceed.

* * *

Remember, as each day goes by it is a day nearer our goal of getting John well again and on the road to a full recovery.

—Jacquie Barcilon

*   *   *

Later that afternoon after the surgery Dr. Skogs met with the Keatings.

"The surgery went well," he began. "We found a lot of dead muscle tissue which we removed. We also had to amputate another five to six centimeters. We still have some room to work with but not much. He will require one maybe two more operations in about two to three weeks time."

The news was good but John was beginning to dread the operations. He worried a lot about them. But for now, he had about two weeks before he had to begin thinking about the next one.

John had begun taking solid food but was not at all impressed with the menu. Swedish hospitals are not unlike those in the United States, and institutional food is "institutional." John was losing weight and not having much success dining on boiled potatoes and fish, especially *Jansson's Frestelse* (Jansson's Surprise), a traditional dish made with potatoes, onions, and anchovies. His mother decided she would augment his diet and began bringing an ice cream-eggnog milkshake every day. John greatly appreciated the supplement.

*   *   *

If thinking and loving help, you can't help improve every day! Remember we're all counting on you and your great spirit to see mending well and soon.

—Maxine Singer

*   *   *

Tuesday, April 28th, as Mike sat in his office reading the morning message traffic, Chief Nowery stuck his head in the colonel's office.

"The mail room just called," George said. "The pouch is in, and there is a package from DIA which looks suspiciously like it might contain a cowboy hat. I'm on my way down there now."

"Great," Mike said as George vanished.

Mike picked up the phone to call Judy.

"Judy, the hat is in. I'll be home shortly, and we'll head to Uppsala."

"Fantastic," she replied. "John will be so happy."

* * *

Keep your head up, keep smiling, and keep laughing—because you do those things better than anyone I know.

—Rob Carter

* * *

The trip to Uppsala was full of joyful anticipation, not unlike parents on Christmas Eve. One of the joys of parenting is Christmas morning when a child, having anticipated Santa's visit, reacts to the sight of the lit Christmas tree and the gifts under it. That moment was reprised when John's parents walked into his room with the cowboy hat. John beamed; his talisman had arrived. The hat gave him a feeling of security. If there had been any doubt in his mind that he was not going to make it, it vanished when he put on the hat. The tale of the hat was one of a well-coordinated effort by several dedicated people. It was symbolic of the love and concern of all of his friends, and it gave all the Keatings an emotional lift.

The next morning when Drs. Hedlund and Skogs arrived with their gaggle of interns and residents, they found John propped up in bed wearing a smile from ear to ear and the cowboy hat perched atop his head.

"Where's your horse?" asked Bosse.

"I fell off," quipped John.

*　　　*　　　*

John I'm so delighted to know that the hat met with your approval—you could only complement it.

—Mary Cronin

*　　　*　　　*

Mike and Judy were overwhelmed when they arrived at their first official function after the accident. The occasion was a dinner party at the home of Poongja and Koeng-ho Chong, the South Korean Military Attaché. The outpouring of support and concern was very emotional. The Chongs were humbled and honored that the Keatings had selected their dinner party for their first official appearance. Many of the guests had been at Storlien and many, like the Chongs, had taken their children on the trip. They were eager to get first-hand information to pass on to their children. The two young Chong girls were permitted to come out briefly to meet the Keatings and to hear that John was doing well, thanks to their prayers and concerns, and that John's friend Animal was keeping him company in the hospital.

*　　　*　　　*

...keep your belief that miracles happen every day in this uncertain world of ours. Our true heartbreaks are in our suffering

over the uncertain events that happen to our children—this is the heritage of a parent.

—Lee King

* * *

Commander Gushaw and the girls had brought John a gag gift, which was a black-lacquered, four-inch cube with a slot in the top where one could put a coin. The coin would rest in this slot and eerie music would begin to play. Then very slowly a trap door on the top of the box would begin to open. Gradually it would open farther and farther as the music continued. Then all of a sudden, without any warning, a green ghoulish hand would come shooting out of the trap door, grab the coin, and disappear back into the box as the trap door slammed shut.

The 79-A nurses thought it to be a rather strange gift. The idea of this ghoulish hand coming out of the box struck them as bizarre, given the fact that John had just lost his entire arm. They seemed to approach the idea and the box itself much like a cat approaches its prey—curious but cautious. Apparently, they collectively accepted the fact that if it did not bother John, it should not bother them. Americans are strange and "the American" was, well, an enjoyable and entertaining challenge. It was not necessary to understand his zest for life in order to appreciate it.

Word of the mysterious "black box" quickly made its way to the other wards and a couple of days later, a nurse from another floor was visiting one of the burn unit nurses. The conversation eventually turned to the "black box."

"Would you like to see it?" she asked.

"Yes, I sure would."

"Come on," she said as they headed for John's room.

"John? Can we come in?" the nurse asked entering John's room. "I have a friend here who would like to see the 'black box.'"

John was sitting up in bed with his cowboy hat on. He introduced himself to the visitor and they shook hands. "If you have a krona, just put it in the slot," John said.

The three waited anxiously as the music began and the trap door began to open. Then in a flash the hand had grabbed the coin and disappeared. All were quite amused.

"John, could I borrow that to show the people on my ward?" the visitor asked.

"Sure," John exclaimed as he handed the nurse the "black box."

Later that evening the nurse, bubbling with excitement, returned with the box and thanked John for sharing it.

After the nurse left, John picked up the box and held it as if judging its weight. *Wow!* John said to himself. *This thing is really heavy. I must have made close to 50 kronor today!*

* * *

> *Basically I just wanted to write to tell you that if you believe that a collective body of people and their faith and love can help you, you sure have it. I have much confidence in you.*
>
> —*Alyson Denny*

* * *

Burn patients frequently suffer severe pain, and John was no exception. In addition, he was also experiencing "phantom pains" associated with amputations. These are pains the patient feels as if they originated in the missing limbs. The severed nerve endings send signals to the brain resulting in the patient experiencing pain. The doctors were having difficulty treating John for pain, and John wanted to decrease the amount of pain medication he was taking because it made him feel depressed and intensified his nightmares, especially the smell of burned flesh and the fear of the unknown.

The doctors discussed the matter openly and frankly with John's parents explaining that one of the medications they initially used was a drug that causes the patient to have amnesia so he doesn't remember the pain. That drug was not an option at this point, they insisted. One of the options they offered was the service of a physician who specialized in the treatment of pain. They were quite guarded in their discussion of this option, because the specialist used hypnosis and the power of suggestion. He was a qualified M.D., an anesthesiologist, and fortunately was located in Uppsala. Their guarded opinion about this form of treatment was a result of the general skepticism held by the medical profession. While Swedish physicians are much more open-minded in this area than their American counterparts, Drs. Hedlund and Skogs proceeded with caution.

The Keatings had no problems at all with this option to the great relief of Hedlund and Skogs. Dr. Hedlund explained that the physician was Dr. Basil Finer, an Englishman, working in Sweden. He was well known and respected in the medical community for his work with pain.

On Saturday, Dr. Finer came to the hospital. He was a short, round man, with a well-trimmed and groomed beard. He reminded the Keatings of the movie actor Sebastian Cabot. His voice was that of a soft baritone—very pleasing to listen to. He was very impressive, and the Keatings hoped he could help.

He spent a little more than an hour with John, taking a case history and simply talking to him. John revealed that his "phantom arm" felt as if it was curled up with the elbow tucked into his side and the hand twisted inward into his shoulder. Under hypnosis, John moved his "phantom arm," stretching it out in front of his body and experiencing relief and comfort. That night he felt much better and his normal sedative was not required.

The next day was Sunday and Dr. Finer returned. This time he spoke to John while John drifted off into a state of calm and serenity. At the end of the session, John awoke and felt very relaxed.

"John, I've made a tape for you. Anytime you feel the pain coming on put this tape on, lean back in your bed, close your eyes and relax, and listen to the tape just as we have done today."

On Monday, John had cut his pain medication in half. Two days later, he no longer required any pain medication.

Later in the week, Dr. Finer returned to visit John to see how he was doing. He was quite pleased with the results. John recognized that the doctor seemed a bit depressed and he questioned him.

"You're a perceptive young man, John," Dr. Finer said.

"You should feel fantastic," John told him. "If I could do for someone what you have done for me, I'd be ecstatic. You should go out and tell people, 'You wouldn't believe what I've done for this poor guy lying in the burn unit up at the Akademiska Sjukhuset!'"

When Dr. Finer departed that day, he felt much better. "The American" had touched him.

* * *

My respect for the Swedish physicians and the British hypnotist is considerable, but then they've got a ***tough*** *and highly motivated young man to work with!!*

—Pete Keating

* * *

Judy sat beside the bed talking with John when one of the nurses walked in and asked, "John, would you like your Mother to take you off the ward for a look around?"

"Yes!" was his immediate response as he sat up in bed.

"She can wheel you downstairs to the main lobby. It will give you a chance to get out of here for a while."

"Great!"

The nurse pushed a wheelchair over beside the bed and assisted him because he still had a catheter. She cushioned his injured leg with a pillow clad in a pillowcase of red, white and blue stripes with white stars in the blue stripes. Judy had brought the pillowcase to him from home earlier. He wore a brown jogging suit jacket over his hospital gown and was tucked in with a hospital blanket. And, of course, his talisman cowboy hat perched atop his head.

Swedes are not prone to greeting a stranger when passing them, not even with a smile or eye contact. So it was an exception for the nurses and doctors to smile at John and say, "Hi!" as they passed in the hall. John initiated many of the greetings, and the Swedes were simply responding even though they had not been properly introduced. While these people were complete strangers to John, many certainly knew of "the American."

When they reached the lobby, people turned to look at John out of curiosity but would quickly look away, always avoiding eye contact. It was simply a natural thing to do. Many had never seen a person in a cowboy hat and he was a curious sight. Several children caught his eye, and John would make a pistol with his forefinger and thumb and pretend to shoot at them. They would smile back at him. On later excursions, John would take Animal, and the puppet mesmerized the children.

* * *

LOVE: 2 cups admiration; 2 cups strength. Stir. Sprinkle with genuine sisterly affection. Serve boiling hot!

—Stephanie Singer

* * *

One day a small package postmarked "United Kingdom" arrived addressed to John. The package contained Paul Brickhill's book *Reach for the Sky,* the story of Douglas Bader, a hero of the Battle of Britain. Inscribed on the inside was:

John Keating—
Good luck!
From
Douglas Bader
25/4/81

Bob Barcilon, while on a trip to London a couple of weeks after the accident, had run into Douglas Bader at the Royal Air Force Club and told him of John's accident. That short encounter resulted in the book being sent to John.

The Douglas Bader story is unique because, in addition to being one of the most courageous pilots in the RAF, he was also legless. It is a story of his ability to conquer his disability.

One of the stories in the book, which John especially enjoyed, was Bader's initial internment as a POW after being shot down over France. In his attempt to bail out, he discovered one of his artificial legs was jammed and he was trapped. With his body half out of the cockpit, he was being battered by the side of the plane as it plummeted downward. Finally, the steel and leather strap of his prosthesis broke and he found himself floating free of the aircraft. He subsequently deployed his parachute but the landing knocked him unconscious. When he came to, three German soldiers were bending over him unbuckling his parachute harness. They carried him to a car and took him to a hospital at St. Omer.

At the hospital, the doctor stitched up a large gash under his chin. As the doctor began to ease Bader's trousers down over his hips, he discovered to his surprise that his patient was a double amputee.

Glancing at Bader, then back at the two stumps and again at Bader, he said in a voice of sober discovery, "We have heard of you."

A few days later while Bader was still in the hospital, a German officer announced to Bader that with the permission of Reichsmarshal Goering, the Luftwaffe had radioed England and offered unrestricted passage for a British communications aircraft to fly at a specific altitude, course and time to St. Omer and deliver a new right leg. Spitfires could escort the aircraft part way and then Messerschmitts would take over. The British could land at St. Omer, hand over the leg, and then depart. The British response was prompt, definite, and to the point. They did not want Goebbels, the Nazi chief propagandist, to reap any propaganda from this "humanitarian gesture" so they replied there would be no free passage or German escort. The RAF would deliver a spare leg in a bomber on one of their normal bombing raids. And true to their word, a British bomber came over St. Omer, the bomb-bay doors opened, a long thin coffin-looking box dropped out, a parachute blossomed, and the spare leg floated gently to the ground amid the puzzled looks of the German antiaircraft gunners.

Meanwhile, Bader was developing an escape plan. He was obsessed with the idea and it consumed him. One night, he slipped away. However, the next day he was recaptured and taken to the headquarters in St. Omer where the Germans took his legs away leaving him helpless, humiliated, and seething. In addition they placed two armed guards to watch him. They were taking no chances! Bader was subsequently transported to Germany and interned in a POW camp where the Germans finally gave him his legs back.

The book was very uplifting and encouraging to John in his recovery. John had a positive attitude from the start and had demonstrated character and tenacity in his battle for survival. The book boosted his confidence that he did have a life after the accident.

* * *

You've gone through the hard part—the remainder is all downhill. You now have the tremendous ability to instill hope in others.
—Teddy Kennedy

* * *

The first week of May had been a busy one for the Keatings. A little more than a week before, Lieutenant Commander Ed Pope, his wife Cheri, and their two little boys had arrived in Sweden. Commander Pope was the new Assistant Naval Attaché replacing Greg Gushaw. On Wednesday, there was a changeover reception followed by dinner at the Keatings' home. Then on Friday, the Gushaw family departed for their new assignment in San Diego, California. It was difficult for the Keatings to bid farewell to the Gushaws because they had been the source of great strength during the past several weeks.

In Uppsala, Friday was also a day of change. One of the nurses came into John's room to inform him that he was being transferred down to the third floor surgical ward. There had been an explosion during a fire in Goteborg and two firemen were critically burned. They were presently being flown to Uppsala, and because there was only one empty room available in the burn unit and they would require two, John was being released from the burn unit. The move was bittersweet. John was sad to leave 79-A and the caring nurses he had come to consider friends, but was pleased that his recovery was far enough along that he no longer needed to be in the intensive care environment.

He had reached another milestone.

"I left behind the beautiful friends in green gowns and blue shower caps whose sterile environment had been my reality for recovery during those critical days," he later would say.

John presented 79-A with a picture book of the United States in which he wrote:

May 8, 1981

79-A

Thank you for the expert attention, the care, and all your warm and smiling faces. When I think back to my stay here, I will always remember the funny things and the beautiful people. I hope you enjoy this book of my country, and I hope you all come and visit me some day. There are so many things to thank you for but the most important is my life. Thank you!

John Keating

* * *

> *You must know we've all been thinking about you—praying for you and aching in our hearts and souls for all you're going through. When the reports finally started coming in that you were feeling better, doing better, flirting with the nurses and all that nonsense, only then did we feel a little better ourselves.*
>
> *—Mrs. Maloney*

* * *

Justin Walker
University of Vermont
Burlington, Vermont

April 22, 1981

Dear John Boy,

I'm sorry I haven't written you sooner, but I have had a hard time trying to put down in writing what I've been feeling. I guess it boils down to: "John, I consider you one of my best friends and if you ever need anything, just yell, and also that I, along with all of your and my friends are behind you all the way." It's strange but I've been thinking about you all the time and all the good times we've had—and listen, we're going to have a lot more!

John, I heard a quote the other day, that I thought you might like to see, it goes: "Nobody says you must laugh, but a sense of humor can help you overlook the unattractive, tolerate the unpleasant, and smile through the unbearable."

But knowing you as well as I do, I bet you are smiling, and making the best of it. I've talked to the boys, Dave, Bill, Mike, & Carl, and hey buddy, we all love you and are going through it with you in our hearts. I sure hope you know that 'cause it's true.

I'd like to repeat what I told you during Thanksgiving break, John—"See it all." Damn, I wish I could talk to you right now. But, I think you know what I'm saying—That we all love you and are praying for you (in our own ways). John, if you can, I would appreciate hearing from you and let me know how you're doing.

Always,
Jud

* * *

Richard S. Wise
New Orleans, Louisiana

April 23, 1981

Dear John,

I was extremely sorry to hear about your accident. As you know, I was wounded in Vietnam and had to spend a year in the hospital as a result. Although my injury was not as serious as yours, the experience gives me an idea of how you feel.

While I was in traction, I tried to stay as busy as possible by reading and exercising the muscles that I could use. And when I finally did get out of traction, I spent a lot more time doing leg exercises than the doctors required. They did not think I would be able to run or play handball again, but I didn't believe them. This gave me a goal to achieve. The striving to achieve this goal kept me from brooding about my situation. If I had brooded I probably would have never achieved it.

You must find yourself a goal to pursue while you are recovering. It doesn't necessarily have to be injury related, it can be anything, mental or physical, but it must be worthwhile so that the striving for it will keep you from feeling sorry for yourself. When you achieve this goal, you will build up your self—confidence, and you'll shoot for another goal even more worthwhile.

Well, here is wishing you all the best of luck and let me know how you're doing.

Dick

* * *

Rob Carter
University of Vermont
Burlington, Vermont

April 24, 1981

John,

Hey, hey dude. Jud told me what happened (Dave called him) and I've been trying to write this letter for a week or so. I'm having trouble figuring out exactly what to say, so I'll keep it short. I feel for you buddy, and I wish it were all a bad dream. I want you to know that even though we haven't seen much of each other since graduation, I consider our friendship still strong. If there's anything that I can do over here, just ask. Even if I can't do anything, we should do a better job of keeping in touch. Just drop me a line if you feel inclined to.

I'm with you all the way Keats, buddy—I'm a damn good listener (or reader as the case may be), **so use me.** *I want to help you in any feeble way I know how. Keep your head up, keep smiling, and keep laughing—because you do those things better than anyone I know.*

My best as always,
Rob

* * *

Mary Cronin
Bethesda, Maryland

April 24, 1981

Dear Colonel and Mrs. Keating,

Our concern for John and interest in his progress continues. Every day begins and ends in prayers for him and with hope that each day is one of improvement. Having your constant love and care is strength to him and his fight to recover is sustaining power for you.

In hopes of expediting the hat to John, through your good friends Suzy Hawley and Dick McHargue, it should be on its way via the Military Attaché mail. I hope this arrangement meets with your approval. Not knowing the delays in regular international mail, particularly for packages, I did not want to risk it being held up in customs or otherwise along the way. My English neighbor says oftentimes her packages to England are two months in arriving.

Bitsy wants very much to come to Sweden this summer and will keep in touch with you as to the best time. I'm having a hard time accepting her being away from home. This past year has been an adjustment for me. I particularly miss her in the afternoons when I see the children come home from school.

Please know you have our support and whatever we can do for you, John, and Joanne will be our pleasure.

In friendship,
Mary Cronin

* * *

Dave Singer
Yale University
New Haven, Connecticut

April 29, 1981

Johnny,

Keepin your head up? Good! Things are getting down to the nitty-gritty. Reading week is just about over and exams are about to start. I've been spending most of my time in the library catching up on reading. I'm in decent shape, but it is still going to be tight at the wire.

Soccer is finished for the spring. I'm not going to get much chance to play in Texas this summer, so I guess I'll concentrate on getting my body back in shape. I'll have two weeks to work out after Bill and I get back from Europe. As it looks now, we leave New York on July 26th and fly to Brussels. Our tentative plan is to go to Paris, then Vienna, Germany, and Stockholm. If you would rather have us come to Stockholm first, we can do that. Since the news here is kinda in bits and pieces, I have no idea how far along you will be back to leading a regular life. If there is any way you can come along with us, COME. Don't worry about putting a strain on our trip. The reason we are going over is to be with you—the rest of Europe is just a side attraction. I'm extending this invitation in the dark about how far along you'll be at the end of July. Anyway, if you don't come with us, we will be in Sweden only in the second week in August.

I'm sure you are beginning to build up Bill and me among the women. Thanks. I expect a letter.

Hello to Mom and Dad. Chin up,

Love,
Starsky

* * *

Suzy Hawley
Alexandria, Virginia

April 30, 1981

Dear John,

What a super letter! We are so flattered that you wrote us so soon. It was wonderful to hear from you—and I loved it that the letter was so honest—not full of a bunch of fakey stuff.

What a man you are! In fact you are just exactly what Dave and I felt you were a year and a half ago. We felt as much that you were sensitive, articulate, and a "thinking" human being—even though you didn't think you were (and still are). I wonder if you can see yourself that way now? Your letter was remarkable for its honesty in dealing with such a terrible and serious accident and its consequences. Yet, the whole tenor of the letter was one of good cheer. Your accomplishment of standing and moving about seems fantastic! Oh, John! How thankful we all are that your life was spared. You have so much to contribute to this world—especially with the attitude you're displaying. I know there'll be down times. You ought to get a tape recorder and put it all on tape so you can get it out of your system.

It is so perceptive to think of your parents. I'm sure they, too, are exhausted. But, you know, you certainly come from sturdy stock—and I don't believe that I've ever known two stronger (inside) individuals or a stronger couple. They're so grateful you're alive! I am certain that the most difficult thing for them is to stand by helplessly as you try to re-order your life. Even though the love and support they're giving you is vital to your recovery, you know they would much prefer to give you an arm and a leg. (By the way, will you ever use that expression again?) And you, John, are so neat to acknowledge their love and caring. God! The sad, little humans I see each day are almost more than a consciousness can bear! Eighty percent of our students come from broken homes—and the number of grade school emotional cripples is overwhelming. Those kids barely have a chance of getting "fixed." I don't really see how our society is to stabilize itself—but that's a much-belabored point. You should read the Alvin Toffler book **The Third Wave.** *Your Mom has a copy.*

I've talked to all sorts of your friends and made lovely new acquaintances…e.g., the Singers and Mrs. Cronin. How they all adore you. Stephanie Singer filled me in tonight on all the hearts you broke at NCS. Shame on you, John! They're all panting for news! (Meanwhile keep those nurses away from my baby…Pete!) Mrs. Cronin has been pleasant…and

I know you talked to them and Bitsy Sunday. How'd that go? What are your feelings these days about B.? Did you ever get things back on the track you wanted? None of my business—but you know I'm damn nosy!

I'm going to send books soon. (Hee hee!) My personal crusade has been to get you reading!!

Keep writing—I'm a pretty good listener.

Love, love, love you,
Suzy

*　　　　*　　　　*

Maxine Singer
Washington, D.C.

May 4, 1981

Dear John,

Since you are now well enough to send welcome letters to your friends, you must also be well enough to put up with the following response: You must learn to spell!!! Now's the time!

From your letter—

recieve: Should be ***receive*** *according to the well-known rule: i before e* ***except*** *after c.*

graph: is reserved for mathematics. If you are an expert it is graft.

(Only a Mom could get away with this.)

Final summer plans fell into place when Amy learned she had gotten the job she wanted. She will be an assistant to the man who constitutes the office of the Jerusalem Post in Washington. She'll have a chance to use her Hebrew and learn a bit about the newspaper business. During most of June and July only Amy will be here—but by mid-August we should all be gathered again.

I am planning on keeping my nose to the grindstone on the book Paul Berg and I are writing. The publisher thinks he will have it on Jan. 1, 1982, but we probably will not make it. Oh well.

Mr. and Mrs. Curran (ex NCS headmaster) bid on our Curacao house at the NCS auction and won it. They go for a week next February and come tonight to hear all about it. Now to the writing!

Love,
Maxine & Dan

* * *

Edward Kennedy
Wesleyan University
Middletown, Connecticut

May 6, 1981

Dear John,

David just told me of your recent misfortune, and I just wanted to let you know how sorry I feel. There are many thoughts that pass through a person's mind when they feel that life has been unfair to them, and it's important that you now realize that although things might seem grim, there is so much to look forward to.

Sitting in a hospital, you probably feel as though you are the only one in the world who has had bad luck. Life has been good to me in many ways, and very bad. It's been good by providing me with many material benefits, but bad because it has been unfair by taking my leg away and giving me cancer. God is also unfair by taking the lives of many of the members in my family. I don't feel sorry for myself, though. I've realized through my experience how much life there really is and how much there is to live for. To be perfectly honest, I consider everything a new challenge. I don't consider myself disabled in the slightest. I've realized just how lucky I've been.

As you make new adjustments, just realize that there are many people that are pulling for you and many people that really care for you. You've gone through the hard parts—the remainder is all downhill. You now have the tremendous ability to instill hope in others.

It's going to be strange for awhile, John. People are going to stare. People are going to treat you differently. But that's their problem, not yours. You can never worry about what others are thinking, or else you'll work yourself into a frenzy.

I am a very happy person with many strong convictions. There is a saying that a person cannot find true humor in life unless he/she has experienced suffering a misfortune. You'll find that it is truly the simple things in life and the relationships you make that make life worthwhile. Life is a series of adapting from one thing to another, which I'm sure you'll agree. Although you might feel that life has been unfair to you, just look at all the people whose lives are benefited by problems beyond their control.

Only you can make the final decision to overcome your disability—but if there is any way I can help, please let me know. Keep it up and go get em!

Your friend,
Teddy

* * *

Dave Singer
Yale University
New Haven, Connecticut

May 8, 1981

Hej!

How ya doin? I'm in a great mood. I just finished my last real exam. I have one left but it's credit/fail and three days away.

I called Teddy the other day. He not only helped me reinforce my positive attitude about you coming back strong but also said he'd drop you a line. We're all pulling for ya. Actually, we are beside you; you are going to be so well off that you won't need people pulling ya. I'm really much better off after your letter arrived. I've read it so many times I think I can recite it off the top of my head. If I hadn't screwed it up opening it, I'd frame the son-of-a-bitch. I'm looking forward to going to Sweden. I know you must feel alone there (you, Joanne, Mom and Dad). But we are all with you all. I wish I could call ya, but don't know how. Next letter give me a number, date, and time for a call.

I figure you're thinking a lot about what you're going to do when you get out of the hospital. Decide what you want to do, and then do it. Don't worry whether you can or can't do something because if I ever hear "can't" from you, I'm gonna nail your ass. I'll stop lecturing.

I'm already psyched about you coming back to the States and being able to visit me up here. I really have missed your friendship and presence this year cause it's been hard adjusting to things and stuff. I haven't been in touch with many people these last weeks because I've been studying so much. I came out okay, I think, but the competition is real tough. Errol and Israel send thumbs up.

We'll be in touch real soon. Looking forward to being with you.

Love ya,
Starsky

* * *

Chapter Four

The Third Floor (May 9–June 15, 1981)

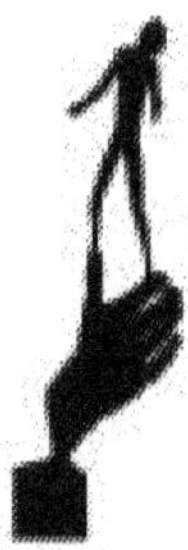

*　　　*　　　*

I love your letters; whenever I feel down I read them, especially the last one. You are the one to be commended; the whole way you take things amazes me.

—Zelda Thomas

*　　　*　　　*

John faced surgery number four the following Monday. Moving from a comfortable and familiar environment, he met a whole new set of caregivers. While the nurses were new to John, "the American" was not new to them. The weekend dragged by with anxiety over the impending surgery but, when Monday rolled around, John had made new friends and was ready.

The surgery went well and consisted mainly of removing dead muscle tissue. He quickly found the nurses on the third floor to be as pleasant and caring as those on the fifth floor. His recovery was rapid, and on Wednesday the Barcilons paid him a visit. The next day Admiral Calle Algernon and Major Erik Hammarskjold drove up from Stockholm to see him, and on Monday the Puntans (Tim and Caroline's parents) came. These visits energized John, as did the letters that continued to pour in from the United States. While his weight had dropped to 134 pounds from 175, he seemed to be gaining strength daily.

For the past several weeks, Torture Lady, the physical therapist, had been working with John to increase his leg strength and balance in addition to his overall physical conditioning. She had him standing unassisted and resisting slight pushes from various directions. She also had him bending down on one leg to pick coins up off the floor. Daily she assigned him a number of sit-ups to do. She would give him a number and he would unfailingly do them, adding five more of his own for good measure. By the end of the summer John was doing 200. John had been progressing well and, as Tuesday arrived, he was looking forward to standing unassisted and embracing his parents with a warm, one-armed hug.

As his parents entered the room, John stood beside his bed with his arm out. "I want a real hug," he said.

His father responded. Father and son embraced in a warm and loving hug. As Mike stepped back, Judy, eager also to embrace John, stepped forward and gave him a firm, emotional bear hug. When she did, John let out a muffled cry of pain and as his startled mother released her hug, John fell back onto the bed. With a pain in his voice, he cried, "Mom, you stepped on my toe!"

Tears of laughter, emotion, and pain were all mixed into one as John exclaimed, "My Mother *Clouseau* and her wooden clogs!"

* * *

I am…thrilled to hear of your progress and to read between the lines the courage, the determination, and the optimism with which you have faced the accident. I knew you would—but it is still good to hear it in your words.

—Mark Mullin

* * *

The nurse John called Tinker Bell was shy and naïve and, of all the nurses, was probably the most uncomfortable with the English language. She had that innocent look and a complexion that telegraphed her bashfulness. John had been removed from all the life support devices, shunts, and catheters save one, the urinary catheter from his bladder. Well over a month had passed and the doctors were becoming concerned. John had been moved from the burn unit to the third floor surgical ward just the week before. The doctors had attempted several times to remove the catheter but the normal urinary functioning had not returned. They had tried everything—giving him water, running faucets, etc. He just could not go. Earlier in the week, the doctors had attempted a cystoscopy in order to determine if there was any type of blockage but were unsuccessful because of the discomfort John experienced as a result of the burns and amputations. They decided to delay the intrusive procedure for a week.

It was Sunday and they were going to try again, before Monday's scheduled cystoscopy, to remove the catheter to see if John could void by himself. John's parents were visiting so they would delay the attempt until after their departure. Tinker Bell had completed her shift in the burn unit and was headed home. Before she left, she stopped by the third floor to check on John to see if he had been successful. Upon noticing his parents, she became very self-conscious and as she asked in her broken English how it had gone, her face began to turn a light shade of pink.

"We haven't tried yet," John explained. "We're going to try after my Mom and Dad leave."

"Oh," she replied turning a full crimson. "Well, good luck with the urine, John."

After his parents left, they removed the catheter, and John was successful in taking care of business. He was now completely on his own. Another milestone.

* * *

While my heart truly aches for each of you, I am so proud to know that a senseless tragedy can unearth such inner power in someone so young—to positively go forward to face and conquer these unpredictable obstacles in his life.

—Pete Armstrong

* * *

One morning as Dr. Hakelius and the gaggle were leaving John's room, one of the young interns remained. After everyone had left, he turned to Judy and asked if he could come back later to talk with John. He told her that he did not understand why John was so positive and indicated that someone very close to him had taken his own life for something far less serious than John's tragic loss. He was quite amazed at John's attitude and wanted a chance to talk to him. Judy told him he was welcome to come back and speak with John.

Later that afternoon, the young doctor returned and found John and his mother alone on the third floor porch. After exchanging pleasantries, the doctor sat down with them.

"John," he began, "I would like you to keep our conversation to yourself because here in Sweden, we are not permitted by law to discuss religion with a patient."

"All right," John responded.

"John, I am looking for knowledge and understanding of your attitude," the intern explained. "Why do you want to live after what happened to you and how have you accepted what has happened? Is it religion? Family? Friends? What?"

He paused briefly and then continued, "John, someone very close to me committed suicide for something a lot less serious than what you are facing and I'm having trouble with it. I don't understand. Are you religious?"

"I believe in God and am a Christian but I don't go to church every Sunday. In fact, I don't go very often at all," John answered.

"What is it then?"

"Well, I guess every living animal has a basic instinct to survive and will fight like hell to live," John replied. "It's a fundamental fact of life. I'm sure you have seen newborns struggle to live. Realizing and accepting that principle, one can conclude it is not an intellectual thing. It is innate in all of us. In addition, I do not believe that God is punishing me for some past sins as some guilt-driven religions might have you believe.

"I believe God is a loving God, full of grace, and not one who goes around punishing people or requiring them to constantly confess their transgressions. I also don't believe He has a requirement to attend church every Sunday or to constantly profess His greatness ad nausea. I believe one can live a religious life and not ever step into a church. Essentially I try to live the Golden Rule. I also don't believe that one religion is any better or worse than any other. Only God can judge that, and personally I think he is very open minded."

John glanced out the window and then continued, "Yes, religion does play a part in my wanting to live because life is sacred, a miracle, and something to be cherished. I believe that. My religion believes that. And so do many others."

"How about your family?" the doctor asked.

"Probably the most important," John answered. "The love I have received my entire life, I sort of take for granted. After all, that is my norm; that's all I know. These past few weeks have made me realize how strong their love actually is. It is the foundation upon which I stand, if only on one leg," he smiled. "I could not have made it if it were not for that love. It has given me the strength to go on, given me energy, vitality. I can feel it."

"You can feel it?" the doctor asked incredulously.

"Yes! It is rejuvenating. I see things more clearly; I can focus better. This also goes to love, concern, and support I have received from relatives, friends, and some people whom I don't even know. You should see the letters I am receiving. Yes, I feel the energy. It is like quenching one's thirst; I physically feel better when my family is with me and after I have read these letters. The pain is not as acute; my fears are not as critical. I am more tranquil."

"Interesting."

"All this probably helps in the healing process too."

"No doubt about it," the doctor answered.

The two continued to talk for quite some time. Finally, the doctor rose, thanking John for his frank and insightful remarks. The young doctor had learned something, something he will carry with him for the rest of his life.

*　　　*　　　*

Rather, it is the ordinary run of us who handicap ourselves so that we never do what we might. John Sharon, in finding his inmost values and reflecting them outward, shows life in its fullness. And so it will be with you, John. How fortunate, how infinitely fortunate, it is for us that you have life and character.

—Ted Eagles

* * *

During a reception at the Swiss Embassy on Thursday night, Bob and Jacquie Barcilon were talking to the Keatings about how well John was doing and how cheerful and positive he had been during their visit the previous week. Judy mentioned in passing that John had expressed a desire to speak with an English-speaking amputee.

The following morning, Sandy, Mike's secretary, called him on the interoffice line.

"Colonel," she anxiously began. "The British Ambassador's secretary is on the phone."

"Colonel Keating," Mike said as he picked up the phone.

"Sir, Ambassador Murray would like to speak to you," said the voice on the other end.

There was a pause. "Colonel Keating, this is Ambassador Murray. Bob Barcilon told me this morning about your son's wish to talk with an English-speaking amputee. I am such a person. Lost a leg on D-Day at Normandy. Would it be all right with you if I went up to Uppsala this afternoon? Say two o'clock?"

"Yes, Sir," Mike replied, still reeling from the shock of having the Ambassador call him directly. "We would be honored."

"Fine. Two o'clock then."

Mike sat there for a moment collecting his thoughts. He looked at his watch. It was only 9:30. Bob must have talked to the Ambassador first thing this morning, he thought. Talk about action!

Mike reached for the phone.

"Judy, I just got a call from the British Ambassador. He wants to visit John this afternoon," Mike said. "He apparently lost a leg at Normandy. That Bob Barcilon is good—really good. I'll be home about 12:30 and we can head for Uppsala."

"That's great!" she said. "John will be so happy and surprised too. See you soon."

When the Keatings arrived in Uppsala, they found John sitting up in bed reading. He was a little startled to see both his parents as normally just his mother made the trip during the week.

"John," his mother began. "The British Ambassador is on his way here to visit you. He lost a leg during the invasion of Europe during the Second World War. He should be arriving about two o'clock."

*   *   *

Some of us are given mountains to climb—damn big mountains—but climb them we will—

—Pete Keating

*   *   *

The third floor staff also had been alerted (probably by the Swedish Foreign Office) that the British Ambassador was coming to visit "the American." As two o'clock approached, John was ready for his visitor.

The Ambassador was ushered into John's room by some hospital official and, after shaking hands with John and his parents, took a seat next to John's bed. Mike and Judy excused themselves and the Swedish official, taking his cue from the Keatings, did likewise. They left John and the Ambassador alone.

"I've heard you've had quite a go," said the Ambassador.

"I sure have, but I'm hanging in there," John replied.

"Lost my leg at Normandy," the Ambassador said. "Was a member of a British commando unit which went in the night before the invasion to mark the beaches. I got wounded in the leg during the invasion and lay on the beach for a day and a half before I was evacuated. There was no way to save my leg so they amputated it. I was 19 at the time, just like you."

"Ever seen a prosthesis before?" he asked.

"No, sir."

With that the Ambassador stood, unbuckled his belt, pulled his trousers down, and then sat back down again. He took his prosthesis off and showed it to John. He demonstrated how his stump fit into the leg and how the leg stays on the stump.

"Nothing too complicated about it. Quite simple actually."

Just then the door opened and one of the nurses walked in to retrieve a thermometer, which had been left on John's nightstand. She didn't bat an eye and the Ambassador didn't skip a beat as he continued discussing his prosthesis.

Here sat the British Ambassador in his shorts, his pants lying on the floor down around his ankles. After she departed, they just smiled knowingly at each other.

"Hopping will become very natural to you," he continued. "There will be occasions when you do not have your leg on and you will find it necessary to hop."

Ambassador Murray smiled and chuckled slightly in anticipation of what he was about to tell John.

"John, after my amputation I was in a hospital back in England. Not long after I had mastered the use of crutches to get around, I, along with several buddies, went down to the local village pub," he said. "We made our way to the bar and all ordered a pint. There was a table open nearby, so we decided to grab it and enjoy my first night out. Because I could not use my crutches and carry my ale at the same time, I decided to carry my crutches in one hand and my mug in the other and simply hop over to the table. Well, after my second hop, I discovered to my horror that my pint of ale was momentarily suspended in the air above the mug. My comrades sat there in shock as the ale hit the floor with a splash heard throughout the pub. The roar of laughter from my comrades soon erased my embarrassment as well as that of the other patrons and everyone had a good laugh. The innkeeper was over to the table in a flash with a fresh pint to the cheers of everyone. To this day, I still chuckle whenever I think about it."

"John," he continued, "you're going to do some dumb things which initially might seem quite natural and logical but turn out to be a disaster. Just remember to laugh it off. At least I've spared you the 'hopping-with-a-beer' disaster."

The two continued to talk for a little more than an hour enjoying each other's company. Finally, the Ambassador said, "John, I've really enjoyed our visit, and I hope we can see each other again when you get out of the hospital."

"Thank you for taking the time to drive all the way to Uppsala to visit and talk with me," John replied.

"My pleasure, John. I want to leave you with one thought, other than not hopping with a beer in your hand," he said. "You have joined a rather exclusive club. You are now an amputee, and with membership comes responsibility. Specifically, if you ever hear of a new amputee, especially one who wants to discuss the amputation or life as an amputee, you drop whatever you are doing and go to him. The shock of becoming an amputee can be devastating, and a person like you who is so positive can make a life-altering difference to someone. You give them all the help you can. The simple fact of letting them know they are not alone is infinitely more important than anything you might be doing."

The two shook hands and the Ambassador departed. As he passed the waiting room, he stopped to tell John's parents that Bob Barcilon was certainly accurate when he told them that John Keating was one great young man.

"My advice is to surround him with good looking young ladies," the Ambassador offered.

Mike and Judy returned to John's room and found that John had hopped unsupervised over to the window to watch the Ambassador enter his silver Rolls Royce and depart. This was the first time he had been out of bed and on his own without the Torture Lady being there.

"That sure was an uplifting experience," John said.

"He spoke very highly of you," his mother replied. "I take it you two had a great time together."

John then related what he had learned about a leg prosthesis and the stories the Ambassador had shared with him. It had been an extremely good afternoon for all of them.

*　　*　　*

I'm really much better off after your letter arrived. I've read it so many times I think I can recite it off the top of my head. If I hadn't screwed it up opening it, I'd frame the son-of-a-bitch.

—Dave Singer

*　　*　　*

After an uneventful dinner that night, John settled back to enjoy TV when there was a sound of a thousand little knocks on the door. Then three of the fifth floor nurses burst in. What a surprise! It had been two weeks since he left the Burn Unit, and he was glad to see some old friends again. He was especially pleased to know that they had not forgotten him.

They were not in their green gowns and shower caps but had their hair down, wearing T-shirts (sans bras), shorts, and looking as beautiful as ever. He was speechless as he sat there soaking up the beauty of these three: the Goalie, Lilla Mor, and Miss Sweden.

"Do you want to go out with us?" the Goalie asked. "We can pick some flowers."

"It will be fun," explained Miss Sweden.

"We'll take good care of you," chimed in Lilla Mor.

John thought he was dreaming and was sure he did not want to wake up because this dream was going to be one heck of a fantasy.

"Sure," he responded, dumbfounded. He had not been away from the hospital grounds since the accident more than six weeks ago.

"Pass me my cowboy hat and let's go!" John said.

The three loaded him into a wheelchair, cushioning his stump with pillows, and headed for the elevators. Down to the first floor and right out the main door they went. The three nurses pushed him along giggling like mischievous schoolgirls.

Eat your heart out James Bond, John thought as "the American" was surrounded by good-looking young ladies just like the Ambassador had advised.

It was a beautiful spring evening, and with the sun lingering in the sky as it does in the higher latitudes, it was magical. The girls picked bouquets of flowers and armloads of flowering branches, depositing them in John's lap. They traveled down cobblestone streets, up over curbs, across gravel paths, and through grassy lawns. Soon the wheelchair was full of flowers and blooming branches. John was hidden in an array of flowers and barely visible. He even had flowers tucked into the band on his cowboy hat.

They entered the park, and as they were proceeding across the grass and down a small incline, one of the wheels of the wheelchair dropped into a small depression, flipping John out of the chair as it tipped over. The girls sat down around John and they all laughed. After a short rest, they righted the wheelchair and attempted to reload John back into it. The Goalie attempted to pull John up by his arm while Lilla Mor braced herself against John's foot so it would not slip on the wet grass, and Miss Sweden maneuvered the wheelchair into position. But as John rose up, his body would twist, since he had no way of keeping his left side from swinging around. This would result in his falling down again. They quickly realized that they needed another person to stabilize him from twisting. A young lady visiting from Luea had been watching them so they enlisted her assistance. With John and the flowers safely back in the wheelchair, they headed for the Castle. As they crossed the sprawling grassy knolls negotiating the rolling terrain, John only fell out of the wheelchair twice more!

It was getting late and John was beginning to feel the cool night air. The sun had finally set, and it was close to 11:30 p.m. when they arrived back at the hospital. The doors were locked. The Goalie rang the third floor nurses' station.

"Third floor!"

"Are you missing a patient?"

"We sure are—'the American'!"

"We've got him down here. Will you ring us in?"

The door unlocked and they were in. After returning John to his room, they departed quietly as John drifted off into a peaceful sleep. The excitement had tired him and he slept soundly. When he awoke the next morning to a room full of flowers, he knew it had not been a dream.

During the morning rounds, the doctors said nothing about all the flowers in John's room. They proceeded as if nothing was out of the ordinary. In a sense, it was business as usual even though the events of the previous evening were the talk of the hospital. The doctors had concluded some time ago that whatever "the American" did was not going to surprise them.

*　　　　*　　　　*

John, you are such a wonder! And I'm sure all who have been around you have gained—by just your determination, strengths, (your antics) and certainly your winning smile.

—Mary Cronin

* * *

John's room resembled a funeral home with its array of flowers, blooming branches, and its aroma of spring. John was beside himself telling his parents about the previous night out, and how enjoyable it had been to see old friends from the fifth floor. They laughed with him as he recounted the events. Hearing of John's falling out of the wheelchair momentarily dampened his mother's enjoyment of the escapade, but the joy and excitement in his voice overcame her anxiety.

After his parents left to return to Stockholm, John felt a little lonely, especially after all the excitement and activity of the previous evening. It was Saturday and nothing was going on.

That sure was fun yesterday, John thought. *I wish I could visit with some of the others from the fifth floor.* The thought lingered for a moment, then he said aloud, "Hum, I'll just grab my hat and go on up there and visit them."

He slipped out of bed and hopped to his wheelchair—wheeled it around and headed out the door. He hit the button in the elevator with his cowboy hat because it was too high for him to reach on the left side. He exited at the fifth floor, proceeded to the burn unit, pushed the button to enter the first set of double doors, and wheeled himself into the "air lock" entryway. The second set of doors presented more of a challenge because he could not push the button and, with only one arm, maneuver the wheelchair through the doors fast enough before they automatically closed. He tried a couple of times unsuccessfully.

Now what to do? He found himself trapped between the two sets of doors. He knew that eventually someone would come along, but how long would that be? After some ten minutes, he decided to try a running start—sort of hitting the button as he was rolling towards the doors. Failure!

He continued to wait. Finally, he decided to try to push the doors open manually using his wheelchair to gain a mechanical advantage. Success at last!

He made his way down to the nurses' lounge where the four nurses on duty were just sitting down to their evening meal. John was welcomed like the long, lost son and was bombarded by questions about his night out. They had a good reunion. One of the doctors came in, greeted John, and asked if the nurses on the third floor knew where he was. He said he had heard that they had "lost" a patient last night.

"I don't know," John said with a smile, evading the question. "I don't know what they know!"

*　　　*　　　*

I was the same age when I made a complete fool of myself. You learn to live with it.

—Douglas Bader to Bob Barcilon

*　　　*　　　*

More visitors, including the Hares, Thomsons, Barcilons, and Julins, kept John away from the self-pity that so often accompanies boredom. John looked forward to the visits, and his stamina was increasing daily. In addition, his spirits always seemed to be uplifted after visitors had been there.

Saturday, May 30th, was a special day. As John and his parents were visiting in his room, a couple of nurses rushed in pushing a table-mounted telephone used by patients to make and receive telephone calls from their room. As one of the nurses was busy plugging the phone in, the other announced, "John, the White House is on the phone."

"What?" John replied, somewhat confused.

"The White House is calling you!"

John picked up the phone. "Hello!"

"Is this John Keating?" the operator said.

"Yes, it is."

"This is the White House switch," the operator said. "Please stand-by. You have a call from Vice President Mondale's residence."

"John!" boomed the voice. "This is Billy. Dave and Carl are here too. How are you doing?"

"Great! What a surprise this is. It's super to hear from you."

They talked for quite some time and John beamed with excitement. Billy Mondale, Dave Singer, and Carl Casimano all talked to John, and his St. Albans' classmates found it reassuring to hear the positive note in his voice. While it is one thing to receive letters, it is quite another to hear a cheerful and confident voice.

When the call finally ended, John was on cloud nine. Dave and Billy would be in Sweden in about 12 weeks. He looked forward to that visit with great anticipation. In fact, he thought about the visit constantly, visualizing what the three of them would be doing. But for now, he had to concentrate on getting better and out of the hospital. His dreams of Dave and Billy's visit did not include their visiting him in the hospital in Uppsala. His mental pictures had him at home in Stockholm.

* * *

Sunday was Swedish Mother's Day. Judy opened a card from John and read:

May 31, 1981

Mom,

Sorry I couldn't get you a real Mother's Day gift. All I have left is my love. I should thank you for your faithful visits and commend you on your strength. All the things I've seen in you help me grow each and every day. I'm glad you're my Mother and I love you every day. I hope you're as happy as I am because it's you who makes me feel this way.

Happy Mother's Day

John

* * *

John was scheduled for his fifth surgery on Wednesday, but it was rescheduled for reasons unknown to him. John was relieved and was looking forward to Friday because he was scheduled to receive a temporary leg prosthesis. It would be fitted and designed to support him at the upper leg and hip region because his stump was far from being ready to receive a prosthesis. This meant he could finally be on his feet and walk again. It would give him some freedom, some independence. He could hardly wait.

On Friday morning, John was ready. When Torture Lady and the technicians arrived with the leg, John was waiting. Because the sides of his leg and his stump were still open and required bandages, the prosthesis was very crude looking. There was a harness ring, padded with leather, which fitted his upper leg at the hip and groin, then two steel bars traveled down to a wooden foot. Along the two bars were straps with belt-buckle latches. It had a hinged knee which had to be locked straight when in use but could be released when John wished to sit down. It was not pretty, but it was functional, and John was eager.

"What do you think?" asked Torture Lady.

"Let's give it a try," replied John.

After strapping the leg on, John stood, first supporting his entire weight on his good leg and then little by little transferring his weight to both. The results of the conditioning and hard work Torture Lady had put him through was evident. He had exceptional strength in his good leg, and the balancing exercises she had made him do had increased his physical strength as well as his confidence and determination. She held his arm for the first couple of steps, and then he was on his own.

John was having the time of his life. Finally, he had to be stopped for fear he was overdoing it. He was disappointed but understood. When Torture Lady did not leave the leg in his room but took it with her, tucked safely under her arm, he recalled the incident when the Germans took Douglas Bader's legs away from him so he would not escape. *Did they think I was going to escape, he wondered. Well, there is always that possibility!*

* * *

> *...everybody is amazed and admiring of his courage and determination.*
>
> *—Ingrid Beach*

* * *

"To John Keating—With admiration of his strength and resolve," was the inscription on one of the several books sent to John by Captain Ned Beach. Mike and Judy had met the Beach family while preparing for their assignment to Stockholm. Ingrid, his charming wife, was a Swedish language instructor at the Foreign Service Institute in Washington, D.C., and Mike and Judy had been her students. John enjoyed the books and was quite honored that the author had inscribed each one with a personal message. John had previously read *Run Silent, Run Deep,* which had been a best-seller and a popular motion picture, and *Around the World Submerged,* the story of the USS Triton, under Ned's command, in her underwater circumnavigation of the earth. The books were a great boost, a blend of action and adventure punctuated with frustration and success with which John could identify. He devoured them.

* * *

We haven't met yet, but our thoughts and prayers have been with you for a long while. We hope to see you Monday.

—Cheri Pope

* * *

The next day was Saturday, and Joanne traveled with her parents to Uppsala. She had graduated from the International School on Thursday evening and had celebrated with some of her classmates on Friday with a swim party at her home. Today she took a short walk with her brother down to the first floor. It made her feel great, and seeing her brother walking again was as exciting as Christmas. The Barcilons came up for a visit later in the day and were also overjoyed to see John walking. It was a milestone, another goal reached. Everyone was very proud.

On Monday, Ed Pope, the new Assistant Naval Attaché, and his wife Cheri and their two boys, Brett and Dusty, paid a visit. It had been difficult for the Keatings to say goodbye to their predecessors, the Gushaws, since they had been so very close during the initial days of this ordeal. Ed and Cheri came up with the boys and joined the Keatings in enjoying a picnic outside on the beautiful hospital grounds. Ed and Cheri added a new energy, instantly bonding with the family. The family aspect of the newly formed friendship was significant in that it established a union which would prove to be a source of strength for all the Keatings in the days ahead. Brett and Dusty were a boost to John and responded to Animal as the children had earlier at Storlien.

Anders Julin also visited John. Anders and Lena had been close to the Gushaws and had heard of John's wish to speak to an English-speaking amputee. Anders was a Lieutenant Commander in the Swedish Navy, but his stepfather was British and lived in England with Anders' mother. He had lost the lower part of his left arm during World War II while serving in the British Navy in the Mediterranean

Sea during the resupply of Malta. He promised Anders he would send a tape with his observations.

* * *

One thing I admire so much about you is your zest for life! I look up to people like you 'cause that's what I want to be like! I also know that you won't let what happened to you interfere with the rest of your life—that's why I think you're so great! YOU AMAZE ME BOY!!

—Dale Banfield

* * *

Your cousin Mike is planning on being with you and family in Sweden in June. I've tried to intercept him in Ireland so he writes first (or phones) so you and Mike Sr. and Judy know he's coming.

—Pete Keating

* * *

It was late in the afternoon and Mike was expecting a phone call from Judy when she returned from Uppsala. John was going to go to the Go Skolen (the Walking School) for the first time and she would be accompanying him. John had spoken of the two prosthetic technicians, Robert and Lennart, and how much he enjoyed them, their upbeat attitude, and their enthusiasm for their work. Mike had just completed reviewing an outgoing report to Washington and leaned back in his chair thinking about his son.

"Colonel Keating, I have a Mike Keating holding on the phone for you," Sandy said interrupting the colonel's thoughts.

"Mike, how are you doing? Where are you?" the colonel asked after picking up the phone.

"I'm at the Sheridan Hotel. How do I get to the Embassy?" asked young Mike.

"Not to worry. I'll pick you up. Will meet you in front of the hotel in about 10 minutes. I'll be in a dark blue Mercedes. How's your trip been going?"

"Wild! Had my money, passport, and VISA card stolen when I was in Dublin. Dad might have told you. Tell you all about it when I see you."

"Good to hear your voice. John will be thrilled to see you. See you in about ten."

As Mike turned into the Sheridan, he had no trouble picking out cousin Mike. He looked as if he had just come out of the wilderness of northern Canada. His bright eyes sparkled from behind his dark beard, and his six-foot stature, broad shoulders, Levis, and sweatshirt set him apart from the businessman crowd.

Mike was the second son of Pete and Sally Keating. Colonel Keating and Pete were first cousins, and during the Second World War when the colonel's father was overseas with the Army, his mother had returned to Neenah, Wisconsin, with her two sons. The two cousins, being only a year apart in age, were very close and spent a lot of time together.

Cousin Mike spent several weeks with the Keatings, and the visit was mutually beneficial. John needed a contemporary with whom to talk, other than just the professional hospital staff, and Mike was perfect because the two had shared the experience of a two-week canoe trip in the wilderness of Canada in 1976. In addition, Mike had lost the ends of two of his fingers in an accident at the Neenah Foundry the previous summer. In relating the story to John, he said everything was fine until the foundry nurse, when calling the emergency squad, used the word "amputation."

"Then my knees just buckled," he confessed.

Cousin Mike accompanied Judy to Uppsala to visit John, and it was during these one-hour drives each way that he processed his feelings about his own accident at the foundry. He explored his goals, admittedly having had no direction in college. Mike became a working member of the family—from doing pool maintenance, to scrubbing and cleaning the boat, to serving and bartending at official dinner parties. He was an asset, and his visit was greatly appreciated.

* * *

Decide what you want to do, then do it. Don't worry whether you can or can't do something because if I ever hear "can't" from you, I'm gonna nail your ass.

—Dave Singer

* * *

Midsummer to the Swedes is second only to Christmas in preparation and anticipation. Celebrating the joy of summer and being outdoors in warm and sunny weather is as fundamental to Midsummer as snow is to Christmas. Maypoles decorated with flowers and flags are raised and become the centerpiece for most of the activities. Relatives and friends gather for dancing, singing, eating, and drinking, as the sun at midnight seems to linger on the horizon and then rises again in its full blazing glory. In modern times, the holiday is celebrated as a three-day weekend falling closest to the summer solstice.

During the morning rounds on the Monday before Midsummer, Dr. Hakelius told John that on Thursday he would be temporarily moved to another ward because of the holiday weekend. The doctor explained that the hospital grants some patients a three-day pass for the celebration, but for those critical patients and those requiring daily medical care, the hospital consolidates the wards in order to provide the maximum number of staff personnel time off to celebrate Midsummer with their families and friends.

"Why can't I have a three-day pass?" John asked.

"Well, John, you require daily medical care," Dr. Hakelius stated. "You need to have the dressings on your leg changed three times a day."

"Couldn't you just send me home with all the necessary medical supplies and have my parents change the bandages?" suggested John.

"I'm afraid not," he said. "The nature of your wounds requires the attention of a trained medical professional."

"How about if I take one of the nurses home with me?" John countered.

The gaggle of doctors now became a little more interested in this banter and the tenacity of "the American." It was not unlike a tennis match with the heads of the doctors going back and forth between Hakelius and "the American" as they volleyed.

"Who do you have in mind, John?" Hakelius asked.

"Isabelle."

"Isabelle Pettersson?"

"Yes!"

The gaggle murmured their approval, as Isabelle was a beautiful blond on the surgical ward to which John was assigned. The momentum had shifted and the gaggle was secretly pulling for John.

"Hum," Dr. Hakelius pondered. "I'll tell you what, John. If you can get Isabelle to accept an invitation to your parents' home for the Midsummer weekend, I'll let you go. We'll provide her with all the necessary supplies she'll need to dress your wounds. This assumes that it is all right with your parents."

"Thanks," John replied with a smirk on his face.

The gaggle approved, somehow sensing it was already in the bag. "The American" had done it again.

It was no surprise to anyone the next day during rounds when John announced to Dr. Hakelius that Isabelle had accepted his invitation. He was going to be spending the weekend at home and sleep in his own bed. What a great feeling!

* * *

We are all dealt a "hand" to play in this game of life and we must play with what we have. It's how we play with what we have that makes the difference in how we live.

—Barbara Leiser

* * *

Around 1:00 p.m. Thursday, John arrived home with Isabelle in her car loaded with medical supplies. It was a grand homecoming albeit for only 72 hours. The Keatings had, of course, met Isabelle on the ward and had been impressed with her. Now they had an opportunity to become acquainted with her in a more informal setting. She was a very quiet, unassuming young lady whose outlook on life was positive. Her blond hair, svelte figure, and comely face made her pleasing to the eye. Her English was excellent, due in part to the fact that she was not only a huge fan of Elvis Presley but also the president of his fan club in Sweden. She was fun and enjoyable to be around and loved to participate in whatever was going on. She was an excellent houseguest, and her role as guest did not interfere with her nursing responsibilities. She made "the American" toe the line and not overdo his freedom. Mike and Judy were not only impressed with her but enjoyed her company very much.

On Friday, the Chongs came by to deliver a cake Poongja had made for John as a welcome-home gesture. They had their two girls with them and came in for drinks. Maria and Bruno Servadei, the Italian Defense Attaché, also dropped in with their children to welcome John home. Both the Chong and Servadei children had been at

Storlien and had been touched by the tragedy. For them to see John and Animal again brought them closure.

John and Animal entertained the children, and everyone sat around the pool, talked, swam, played bocci, and had refreshments. The fact that John did not have an arm or walked stiff-legged did not seem to bother the children as John joined in playing bocci with them. It was a delightful, impromptu afternoon.

The Keatings had invited Robert and Jackie Barcilon over for a Midsummer dinner. It was a small intimate gathering, served outside, with John, Joanne, Isabelle, and cousin Mike. Mike also doubled as the bartender. It was a pleasant and joyful evening for the Keatings, having John home and being able to share this time with the Barcilons who had been so supportive.

Cousin Mike returned to the United States the next week to continue his education at the University of Wisconsin. He also carried back to all the Wisconsin family members the message that John and his family were not only coping but also inspiring those around them.

* * *

...no matter what else you have lost, I hope you don't lose all your passion for things and living...

—Susy Cromwell

* * *

The Wednesday following Midsummer, John had his fifth surgery. He had made it perfectly clear when he first met Dr. Finer that even though the doctor considered him an excellent candidate for hypnosis, he would never consider undergoing surgery under hypnosis. John was not too enthralled with the idea of being completely "knocked out" either. Dr.

Hakelius had suggested they might try a spinal block to just anesthetize the lower half of his body. John agreed and that was the procedure used.

In recounting the surgery, John related, "Everything went well until they started to saw another two centimeters off the stump. The sound of the saw was chilling. I got them to sing *Helan Gor,* loudly I might add, to help drown out the noise of the saw. They were very accommodating, and I joined in singing along with everyone else as the saw did its work." (*Helan Gor* is a Swedish drinking song that translates "The Whole Thing Gone.")

Dr. Hakelius reported to John's parents that they had to remove another 2.5 centimeters from the leg, but he believed there was enough of a stump remaining to use a below-the-knee prosthesis. He also told them that they were able to close the skin around the stump.

John could not come home the following weekend, but the next weekend he and Isabelle arrived on Friday. Judy's birthday had been the day before, but the family had delayed the celebration so John and Isabelle could be there. They celebrated at home with a fine dinner, ice cream, and cake.

Saturday was the Fourth of July and the Keatings hosted a small party including the Soderholm family (Swedish neighbors and close friends) and the Barcilons, along with their daughter Nichola, who was visiting from England.

* * *

> *You must find yourself a goal to pursue while you are recovering. It doesn't necessarily have to be injury related, it can be anything, mental or physical, but it must be worthwhile so that the striving for it will keep you from feeling sorry for yourself. When you achieve this goal, you will build up your self-confidence, and you'll shoot for another goal even more worthwhile.*
>
> —*Dick Wise*

* * *

Monday, June 13, was John's 96th day in the hospital. During rounds that morning Dr. Hakelius announced that he was going to release him from the hospital on Friday.

"What do you think of that, John?" the doctor asked.

"Not much!" John replied disappointedly.

The gaggle stirred uneasily as they collectively shifted their weight from one foot to the other.

"What do you mean, John?" Dr. Hakelius asked somewhat surprised. "Aren't you ready to leave? You've been asking almost daily when we were going to release you."

"Well," John said. "I want out on Wednesday this week; Thursday, the absolute latest."

"We can't do that John," Dr. Hakelius explained. "We only release patients on certain days. Our out-processing and administration paperwork is geared to specific days in order to be more efficient. And those two days are not 'release days.'"

"Doctor, since I first arrived, I have been told, in fact encouraged by the entire staff here to set goals for myself," John explained. "'This is part of the recovery process,' you've told me. Well, one of my goals, as you well know, was to get out of the hospital before 100 days are up. Thursday is day 99. I've done everything you have asked of me and more."

"That's our system, John," the doctor said as he and the gaggle departed.

Dr. Hakelius could not have missed John's disappointment, nor could he have missed the first glimpse of despair he had ever seen on "the American's" face. The atmosphere was thick and tense.

The next morning when the gaggle arrived, the atmosphere had not improved. The interns and residents looked serious and very businesslike as they moved around John's bed.

"John," Dr. Hakelius began "how are you feeling today?"

"Okay, I guess," John answered curtly.

"Good enough to go home tomorrow?"

"Whoop!" John exploded, startling the gaggle.

He was sitting straight up in bed pumping his arm up and down with excitement. The gaggle was inwardly cheering right along with him. He was going to make his goal! He was being released on day 98!

* * *

Life is too important to be hindered by the trials. I try to learn through the pain, joy, disgust, encouragement. Don't give up whatever you do.

—Shalini Amerasinghe

* * *

The Keatings picked John up at the hospital and received detailed instructions about visiting the local district nurse in Djursholm daily to have his dressings changed, appointments at the Go Skolen, and follow-up appointments with Dr. Hakelius. It was an emotional departure for, after all, John had spent some 98 days there and these were the people who had nursed him back to health. They also were saddened to see "the American" go because he had been one of their success stories. They, along with John's spirit and determination, had been a winning combination. For John, the future was out there for the taking, and for them it was back to the job of trying to save shattered lives and bodies. Certainly many must have thought, *Think of the numbers we could save if they only had "the American's" heart and will.*

* * *

Have a good day. Smile for me!!!

—Susan Lane

* * *

Jeff Ingraham
St. Albans School
Washington, D.C.

May 11, 1981

Dear John,

I'm not sure really how to begin writing this letter because I didn't know you that well when you were at St. Albans. When I heard what happened to you, I was totally blown away. I felt so bad, everyone did. You have a lot of friends here who care about you. And when I see what you must be going through, it makes me think about whether even I have a right to give you any consolation.

I lost my leg to cancer when I was in the eighth grade. The only thing I could think about was that I would be handicapped for the rest of my life. It was really frightening. But then I realized that at least I was alive, and as the months went by, it was something I came to accept.

The first stage of making a new leg for me came with a cost. It had a steel pipe attached to a simple knee joint mechanism. One thing that you will experience is phantom pain. It's like an itching or burning sensation coming from a specific point where your limb used to be (your toes, for example). It's pretty bizarre but it becomes much more occasional and less intense as time passes by. My amputation was four years ago and I rarely experience phantom pains at all.

I just wanted you to know that I can relate to what you're going through. It can be such a bitch at first but you can't let it slow you down.

I had a difficult time learning to walk with an artificial knee joint at first. From what I understand, your amputation was below the knee and the fact that you have your knee joint will make things easier for you. As far as your arm is concerned, I know nothing about arms. As with the leg,

I'd think you'd have to wait for the swelling to go down before getting fitted with anything permanent.

You learn a lot about people but more importantly, you learn **a lot** *about yourself. That in itself is rewarding. I consider myself a strong individual; from what I've heard about you and the way you are, I think you will come out of this a stronger person yourself. There is so much you can do! I hope at this point things are going all right for you. I think about you a lot. Write back if you get a chance, I'd like to hear from you.*

Take care,
Jeff

* * *

St. Albans School
Mount St. Alban
Washington, D.C.

Headmaster's Study

May 14, 1981

Dear John:

How wonderful it was to have your great letter arrive today! Of course, I am terribly touched and pleased that you have felt the concern and love that so many at St. Albans are sending your way. The bond you spoke of between graduates and the whole community is the most wonderful thing anyone could say about the school. But I am even more thrilled to hear of your progress and to read between the lines the courage, the determination, and the optimism with which you have faced this accident. I knew you would—but it is still good to hear it in your words.

As a matter of fact, when word of your accident spread at school, several people said to me that there was no one in the Class of '80 who would be stronger or better able to bounce back from such an ordeal than John Keating. The other thing being said around school is that you are already flirting with the Swedish nurses! That doesn't surprise me either, and I worry more about them than about you if you are, indeed, in the hospital two more months.

As you know, we have two new lacrosse coaches and until they ran into a very tough Landon team, they had the spring season going extremely well. That reminds me to tell you that when I first spoke to the student body about your accident, I told them that my most vivid image of you was your charging down the lacrosse field with a feather in your helmet, looking absolutely ferocious and terrifying. Then you walked over to the sidelines where you were as gentle and kind to Kevin Mullin as any person could possibly be.

It appears we have survived (narrowly) senior prank with a minimum of problems. But maybe I am holding my breath too soon.

Do give my best to your parents. Thank you for the wonderful thoughts you expressed in your letter. I did have to laugh at your concern about spelling! I guess one can never escape from the influence of the St. Albans English Department. Hang in there, and do know that you continue to be supported by the love and prayers of so many people at St. Albans, and very much mine.

Sincerely yours,

Mark H. Mullin
Headmaster

* * *

Edward P. Eagles
St. Albans School
Washington, D.C.

May 17, 1981

Dear John,

I have wanted to write you very much, but I have delayed until I could enclose the final issue of the "News," just printed. You will notice the boys' concern for you in a short piece on page two.

Your dreadful accident, and indeed the shootings of our President and the Pope, force the realization of how precious life is. When I try to put myself in your place, I realize you must have not only physical pain but moments of profound depression. But the important thing is that you have your life and that you are going forward to make a contribution with it—almost certainly a deeper, richer contribution to other people than you would otherwise. How ironic and yet how infinitely important! You and I, as sons of military officers, have each wondered how we would act under fire in combat. But gallantry comes in unexpected ways, even unrecognized by the hero, who does what he does because that's the way he is.

Do you remember a chapel talk last year by John Sharon? It made a profound impression on me. He was speaking about forms of character and courage and it seemed to me he exemplified his theme. When I first saw him as a third former, I was taken aback by his deformed limbs and staggered walk. He was handicapped, so I thought. Then I became aware of his rich personality and his powers of leadership. (Remember his pushing for a booth at the Flower Mart?) **Where** *is his handicap? Rather, it is the ordinary run of us who handicap ourselves so that we never do what we might. John Sharon, in finding his inmost values and reflecting them outward, shows life in its fullest. And so it will be with you, John. How fortunate, how infinitely fortunate, it is for us that you have life and character.*

I want very much to see you when you return to the States. In the meantime, in another letter I'll tell you of the spring antics of this year's seniors. You can see from the cartoon also on page two that "Boomer" Brown got himself in the middle of the intended spring prank. But that's a story for another letter.

Your friend,
Ted Eagles

Keating Recovering

John Keating, member of the class of 1980, recently suffered a tragic accident outside Stockholm, Sweden. As a result of injuries incurred when he touched a high voltage power line, John's left arm and left leg had to be amputated. He has made a remarkable swift recovery, and has already learned to maneuver in a wheelchair. John is staying at Uppsala Hospital, located just outside Stockholm. He may leave the hospital as early as this week, but does not plan to return to the United States until June 1982. Several months from now, John will go to Wiesbaden, West Germany, for further treatment and fitting for an artificial leg. Until then, John can be reached through his father. Please send all letters to c/o Colonel Michael R. Keating
American Embassy

Strandvagen 101
S-115 27 Stockholm, Sweden
The "News" and all of us at school wish him the best.

(The St. Albans News, May 15, 1981, issue 9, Volume LX, p.2.)

* * *

The Piggott Orthopedic Clinic, PA
333 West Palmetto Street
Florence, South Carolina

J. BURR PIGGOTT, JR., M.D. ORTHOPEDIC SURGERY

May 20, 1981

Mr. John Keating
The American Embassy
Strandvagen 101
S 115 27 Stockholm, Sweden

Dear John:

I have just read of your recent serious accident in the May 15 issue of the St. Albans News and have also received a separate letter from your friend, Mr. Ted Eagles of St. Albans, asking that I write to you. I am a graduate of the class of 1940 at St. Albans, having put in 8 years as a student at the school and loving every minute of it. I, of course, graduated some 13 years before your father graduated in 1953 and thinking about it, I probably am old enough to be your grandfather at this point. My main and present situation, however, is that I am presently a paraplegic, confined to a wheelchair after a boating accident some 11-plus years ago in 1969, that left me paralyzed from mid chest downward.

First, let me give you my deepest sympathy and then a few words of encouragement. I know that you are depressed and this is perfectly normal and natural and will pass rather rapidly as you get up and going. Work with your physicians, be attentive and appreciative of their recommendations and instructions and they will respond in kind. Let people help you—I don't mean the hospital staff, but folks with which you later come in contact; you will be surprised at how many folks really do want to help and how many fine people there are in the outside world. I have long since learned that many really want to help in little situations and it almost makes their day more pleasant to be of some assistance to those of us who can't quite do it all on our own.

Try to find that wherein your interest lies and what work you really enjoy doing. My greatest asset has been my family support and being in a field of work that I most thoroughly enjoy, almost as a hobby, as opposed to drudgery and which is definitely rewarding. Your next few months will be somewhat tough, but no one has yet told me that life was a guarantee of ease and we all have our ups and downs. Just hang in there and give it your best shot and I am sure you will come out a winner in the long run.

With warmest regards, I am

Very sincerely,
Burr Piggott

*   *   *

Robert Paul Gabriel
Washington, D.C.

May 30, 1981

Keats:

I'm not too good at writing letters like these, but would like to extend my deepest sympathies to you and my hopes for your speedy recovery. I'm sure many guys (in our class for instance) would "roll over and play dead" and isolate themselves with their own misery if this had happened to them, but not you. You're tough and resilient, yet fun loving and easy-going (a rare combination). I know you'll pull through with flying colors.

On a separate note, I understand you'll be in Wiesbaden for treatment this summer. I'll be continuing my studies at the Goethe Institute in Freiburg (in southern Germany near the Swiss border) from June 9 – August 5, and might travel thereafter. It would be fun if I could come visit you. Write or call me in Freiburg to let me know of your summer whereabouts.

Hope to see you.

All the best,
Bob

*　　　*　　　*

Dale Banfield
Holton-Arms School
Bethesda, Maryland

June 3, 1981

Dear John,

I was so happy when I got your letter I almost started to cry. You sound like you're doing well and that's great. Dave Singer called me yesterday and told me he'd talked to you the night before. He said you are now bombing around in a wheelchair and driving all the nurses crazy! That doesn't surprise me at all!

I only wish I could come see you in August with David. I'm going to Sweet Briar College next year. It's an all girls' school just outside Lynchburg, Va. I don't know if you knew I was a twin, but my brother is going to Washington and Lee University in Lexington, Va., so he'll only be about 45 minutes away, which is pretty good.

Well, I graduate at 10 a.m. tomorrow morning! I can't believe I'm getting out of high school! I remember last year—I didn't make it to your graduation because the Holton prom was the night before and I didn't get in 'til 5:45 and was in no mood to get up and be at STA by 10! I'm sure it was a beautiful graduation though. I've been invited to graduation this year by Brian and Earnesto! Anyway, would you believe it's supposed to rain tomorrow? I'm so mad I could cry—Dave said he'd try to come—I only wish you could be there also—if you were—I'd make sure I threw my bouquet of flowers right at you! I'm going to sign off now 'cause it's getting late and I have a ***hell*** *of a day ahead of me tomorrow—I'll write later and tell you about graduation! Take care.*

All my love and God bless,
Dale

* * *

St. Albans School
Mount St. Albans
Washington, D.C.

Headmaster's Study

June 12, 1981

Dear John:

Graduation was on June 6th and as always it was an impressive ceremony. This year, however, it was a bit unusual. As you know, the Bishop's son was graduating and as each boy came forward to receive his diploma and shake the Bishop's hand, he gave the Bishop three jellybeans. Now anyone can deal with three, or six, or nine jelly beans but after about the fifth graduate had come forward the Bishop was in trouble. Of course, he and I were in robes and so had no pockets. The Bishop handed me a few, then handed a few to the verger, and a few bounced down the stairs. But when Tommy Walker came forward to get his diploma the Bishop poured all the jellybeans into his pocket. It was a joke that everyone enjoyed. I don't know if Tommy ever got that sticky mess out of his pocket!

It is quiet now in School but a week from now all the summer programs will begin, and things will be wild as usual.

I do hope you continue to make progress. Very best wishes.

Sincerely yours,

Mark H. Mullin
Headmaster

*　　　*　　　*

Mary Cronin
Bethesda, Maryland

June 21, 1981

Dear John,

'Tis a quiet Sunday night for a change so I'm going to devote my time to answering your letter and just saying "Howdy." Bee has left a void in my life by taking off for the summer. Seems her vacation at home was just too short. She stirs up so much activity when she is home and gets me into forward gear then ups and leaves. I deflate faster than I inflate. Anyway, I loved the short time I had with her but feel the challenge of being a camp counselor will offer a new horizon. Had she been able to make the trip to Sweden I was seriously thinking of tagging along—another time maybe.

Well, I hear you are up and about, possibly going home this month. John, you are a wonder! And I'm sure all who have been around you have gained—by just your determination, strength, (your antics) and certainly your winning smile! You'll have much to tell when we all meet in the near future.

I wish I could tell you how wonderful Washington is these days but you know there wouldn't be an ounce of truth in that statement. Certainly we've had rain every day since May 1 and the day I put Bee on the plane to Wisconsin it was 100 in the shade.

John, I'm so delighted to know the hat met with your approval—you could only complement it.

John, much love to you from all the Cronins, Bee's Aunt Katie and my Mother—they are always asking about you and asking to send their love. Bee will make it over yet so please don't give up on her. Give my best to your parents.

With fondness,
Mary Cronin

* * *

Thomas P. Liddy
Fort Washington, Maryland

June 21, 1981

Dear John,

The year for me kinda sucked, but I loved it anyway. The swimming team was 9-1, that ain't bad, but I didn't do very well. I got really sick right before the Metro's and lost 17 pounds. I had fun though. My grades sucked. I graduated…and didn't get into my first choice college (worst of all I only applied to one).

I will be taking a semester off. This summer (Aug.) I'm going to do some traveling. I'm going to Indonesia, see India, to Egypt to see Dudley and, if you'll have me, to Sweden to see you. I'll be coming to Sweden near the end of August. Write me and let me know all the garbage I have to know, like where you live and how I get there, and what shots I need, and water that's good to drink, and how many mosquito nets to bring, and precautions to take, and don't let your parents read this letter or they'll think I'm as crazy as you.

Everybody over here has been thinking about you. Even people who didn't know you. We all love you. I heard Dave and Wiggy will be visiting you too, maybe I'll run into them, but I don't really know yet.

Fight like hell, buddy. You know as well as everybody and anybody that you're worth it.

Take care,
Tom

* * *

Dave Singer
Washington, D.C.

July 1981

Keatings,

Here is our schedule. Sorry I haven't been much of a pen pal but I've been working 15 hours a day so I can come see all of you. Other than work, everything is great. I've seen some mighty exciting pictures in ***Playboy****. (John explained them to me.) But the one of John had to be one of the most exciting even though I'm sure we all agree in a different way. I actually needed a picture of John, because I needed it to put next to my picture of Joanne. Could use one of Mom and Dad too.*

Johnny,

Great to hear you're throwing the disc around! You'll have to teach me how to throw when we get there. I never could throw those plastic-paper dinner plates.

William's fishing in the Artic Circle with his folks. He finally got his driver's license. Thank God!

See y'all real soon,

Love,
Starsky

* * *

Barbara Leiser
Dallas, Texas

July 12, 1981

Dear Judy and Mike,

I talked to Patti Curtis last night and she told me about the tragedy that happened to your boy. I am so sorry! I wish there was something I could say to you that would help. Just know that I have you in my heart and my prayers.

…

How is your daughter? I have thought of you all so often. How is your son? Does he have a positive attitude about his future? How are you holding up? You are THE most important factor in his attitude. If he sees pity in your eyes, he'll have a tendency to feel sorry for himself. If he sees love and courage and confidence in him—in **his** *being able to handle* **his** *adversity—then he'll be able to reflect it in showing you how he can grow and build from here and now.*

We are all dealt a "hand" to play in this game of life and we must play with what we have. It's how we play with what we have that makes the difference in how we live. I found this out very late in life. Let's say I ACCEPTED this late in life—I had heard it but wouldn't accept it. I kept living for tomorrow—a tomorrow I finally realized would never come—that it would always be TOMORROW and if I wanted to live, I had to LIVE TODAY—today is all we have now, and we must live it now. Yesterday is gone, finished, and tomorrow may never come and we certainly can't control it so all there is is NOW and we had best do, live, love, and enjoy today. On my deathbed I do not intend to look back on my life and say, "Oh, God, why didn't I do this like I wanted to—I always wanted to do that—SOMEDAY—and now it's someday and I never did." I'm going to live today like it is the last day of my life.

Mike's accident was the beginning of the stirrings within me. I began to see life for what it was and not for what I wanted it to be. It's really when I first started learning how to live and be happy—content in me. I accepted what I was and what I had to work with—this was me—no more and no less—had to work within this framework. We only get as far as we strive to get—no one else can do it for us nor give it to us. This was the beginning of my life. I hope that maybe this might help you and your son.

My love,
Barbara

* * *

Susy Cromwell
Rockville, Maryland

July 14, 1981

Dear John,

I was talking to Justin at a party last week and I told him that I wanted to write you but that I wasn't sure what to say, or if you even wanted to get letters from girls who used to lust after you. So we (Justin and I) in our respective drunken states decided I should write you an incredibly pornographic letter, make lascivious allusions, and try to seduce you cross-continently by mail. I don't think I'm quite capable of such an effort even wasted, and now I'm sober, but I decided to write you anyway.

When I first heard about your accident I was told some outrageous tale, that you were in a train wreck, and one of the few survivors, that you pulled yourself out of the train and grabbed a power line and lost your arm and your leg. When I was finally told by someone that you were drunk and running along the top of some boxcars when it happened, I decided that sounded a little bit more like you. Well, however it did happen, John, I'm sorry. I hope you are recovering as well and as fast as you can. I wish that I knew how you were feeling about yourself and what happened now, and had these perfect words of wisdom or some such crap to make you feel good inside your heart and your head. But I'm not wise, and I don't know if you really want to hear anything from me.

As little as I knew you our junior and senior years, it just seemed to me that you were very much alive, and like a lot of other St. Albans students I knew, too much alive for those surroundings. Even after an eye-widening year of "college life in the 1980's," I must say that you are still the most seductive young man I have ever met. Seduction is a lost art, it really is, and very few people make the effort to be good at it, and I hope that you don't stop because it would make me sad if you did. There, that is as pornographic as this letter is going to get. I guess I'm trying to say that, no matter what else you have lost, I hope you don't lose all your passion for things and living, although passions sure do take a beating nowadays.

I'm working with a landscaping company, and volunteering downtown at a place called ***Bread for the City****. The landscapers I work with (that means YARD WORK) include a male-chauvinist-bible-waving-Xstian-Italian who is my foreman, who can't stop (1) saying that he isn't prejudiced against women, and (2) making comments about their legs, breasts, asses or driving ability, and a crazy vegetarian-Jamaican who does things like tell Judy Odell and me that we are beautiful (and other things) when we are hauling branches, sweating like pigs, and scratching our poison ivy. The whole scene is a little unbelievable, and makes me laugh hysterically.*

Bread for the City *is a small organization on 14th Street, which gives free food and clothing to people who live in NW D.C. and are over 60 or disabled or have dependent children living with them. Between the prostitutes, drunks, transvestites and fights, I am seeing a little bit of inner city life, along with wondering about the exact effect that social programs have in a society, etc.*

Next week I'm going to go to Seattle, Wash., to hike with my sister on the Pacific Crest Trail or in the Cascades. I can't wait to get out of this disgusting Washington, D.C., humidity. Then I am going to go to Squam Lake, N.H., to stay with my family in our house.

This letter is going to end now. I hope you will write me back sometime, because I won't write back unless you do, probably. Please tell me how you are doing, and what you'll be doing. I would like to know.

Take care,

Susy

* * *

Chapter Five

Suzy's Visit (July 16–July 31, 1981)

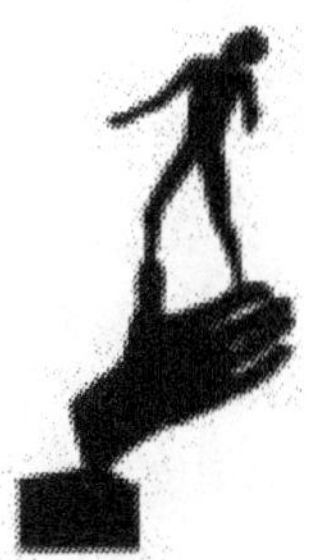

*   *   *

I have admired the sailboats I sent you for well over a year. It gives me such a thrill to send them to my beloved friends. It further connects the families in my heart because I always remember the two silver sailboats that Mummy had on a circular mirror on our dining table when I was very young. And, of course, they carry the significance of the wind being back in the Keating sails.

—Suzy Hawley

*   *   *

Suzy Hawley sat patiently in the Pan American preloading area at Dulles Airport. Her flight to London, with a connecting flight on British Airways to Stockholm, had been delayed again. Here it was almost 10:30 p.m. and the flight had already missed its scheduled departure time by more than three hours.

Her thoughts drifted back some 12 years, as they often had in the past few months, to when she and her two boys had been neighbors of the Keatings while her husband Dave was in Vietnam. She had met Judy, John, and Joanne a few months before Mike returned from his tour in Vietnam. The two women had developed a strong bond and it carried over to the rest of the family.

John was a 7-year old at the time, and Suzy was instrumental in stirring in him an interest in reading. John was a little older than her Pete, and Mark was just a toddler, but, somehow, living in a small housing development nestled in the pine trees of the Black Forest just outside the United States Air Force Academy in Colorado, was a magic environment in which all the kids, plus several dogs, always seemed to travel and play together. The Keating kids, the Hawley kids, the Snowaert kids, the Sandfort kids, *et al.*, enjoyed each other and played well together. It was an idyllic time for the children even though the mothers were under the constant stress of having husbands in Vietnam.

"Your attention please," blasted the loudspeakers. "The Pan Am flight to London is now ready for boarding."

Suzy's thoughts were instantly catapulted back to the present as she collected her belongings and moved to board one of the large people movers unique to Dulles. Suzy looked at her watch. It was after 11:00. *There is no way I can make my connection in London. Hope they can get me on another flight,* she thought.

* * *

The excitement grew with each mile as the Keatings approached Arlanda. They knew the road well because Stockholm's international airport was a little less than halfway to Uppsala. Suzy's flight was due to arrive at noon and after parking the car, they hurried into the terminal with great anticipation. The British Airways jet from London pulled into the gate on time and the passengers began deplaning. Necks were craning trying to get a glimpse of Suzy—but no Suzy! The plane emptied and still there was no Suzy.

Mike checked the information Suzy had sent them. "This is the flight all right," he declared. "Do you think she could have missed her flight?"

"Let's check on when the next one is due in," Judy suggested.

They walked over to the British Airways counter. "Do you have another flight from London today?" Mike asked.

"Yes, sir," the attendant answered. "We have one due in about an hour."

"I guess we might as well wait to see if she's on that one," Judy suggested.

"Good. But if she's not, we probably should go home in case she is attempting to contact us," Mike suggested.

The next flight arrived and no Suzy. Everyone shared in the disappointment, which made for a long drive home. The anticipation of seeing Suzy had been building for days so the letdown was especially hard. However, they took comfort in knowing that Suzy was out there somewhere trying to get to Stockholm and the Keatings' house. Their place was at home near a phone so she could call them.

*   *   *

Suzy finally arrived at Arlanda at 7:15 p.m. She was excited but her thoughts were on calling Mike and Judy. She held out little hope that they might be there to meet her. After all, she was more than seven hours late. A soon as she could get to a phone, she would give them a call.

After claiming her baggage and clearing customs, she headed to a public phone and fumbled through her purse looking for their telephone number.

I know that I have that number in here someplace, she thought. *Now where could it be?* She continued to rummage in her purse.

She then attempted to visualize the piece of paper upon which she had written it. She saw it on the refrigerator in her kitchen at home being held in place by one of those cute little magnets. *Ah, nuts,* she thought. *I've left it at home. I forgot to take it off the refrigerator. No problem. I'll call the operator.*

The operator spoke English so that was a great relief, but she told Suzy that Colonel Keating had an unlisted number, the American Embassy was closed, and suggested she not call the Embassy emergency number. *Now what?* She thought.

"Colonel Hawley, will you accept a collect call from Stockholm, Sweden, from a Suzy Hawley?" the international operator asked.

"Yes, I will," he answered.

"Go ahead, please."

"Dave! My plane was over seven hours late, Mike and Judy aren't here, and I have cleverly left their phone number on the refrigerator. Would you please give it to me?"

"Sure. How was the trip?"

"Horrible! Didn't get out of Dulles until 11:30 and, of course, missed my connection in London. But I'm here now and excited about seeing the Keatings.

Dave gave the phone number to Suzy.

"Thanks, Dave. Love you."

"Say hello to everyone for me."

"I will. Bye."

"Bye."

*　　　*　　　*

The phone rang about ten minutes into dinner.

"Hope that's Suzy," Joanne said.

"Hello."

"Mike, this is Suzy!"

"Where are you?" he asked giving a thumbs-up signal to the rest of the family.

"Arlanda," she answered. "We were late getting out of Dulles, missed my connecting flight in London, and had to call Dave to get your phone number because I left it at home."

"Sit tight. We're on our way. See you in about 30 minutes."

"Great! Looking forward to it."

The family abandoned the table and headed for the airport.

The table must have made quite a sight for the Thomsons who had dropped by to welcome John home. They had rung the bell at the front door but no answer.

"They have got to be here," Bob said. "Mike said they were not going anywhere tonight."

"Lets walk around to the front porch, they could be sitting outside," Mary suggested.

When they could find no one, they looked through the floor-to-ceiling windows that stretched across the entire front of the house. The dining room table was completely set for dinner. In fact, they noticed that the glasses were partially full, food was on the plates, and food was even stuck on a couple of forks. It was a curious sight. It appeared as if they had simply disappeared into thin air, right in the middle of dinner. The scene fit a scenario of an alien abduction!

* * *

Suzy was greeted with hugs and kisses from everyone. She was glad to finally see the Keatings and overwhelmed to see John out of the hospital. John being home was a very special surprise for her.

"John," she said hugging him as if to validate that he was really alive. "When did you get out?"

"Yesterday!" John exclaimed. "I told the doctors Suzy was coming so they had to let me out."

"I had no idea you would be home. This is so great!" she exclaimed as she hugged them all again.

It was a special moment for all. Suzy felt reassured that the family was doing okay and coping. It gave her a tremendous sense of relief. After all the worry and concern of the past several months, she felt comforted. It was as though a heavy burden had been lifted from her shoulders. She quickly forgot the problems she had experienced on her trip and how tired she was. She was now basking in a glow of contentment.

"Oh, you guys look so great! I love you all!" she said bubbling with excitement.

The Keatings felt the same emotion. Suzy epitomized all the hopes and prayers of the many friends who had written. Here she was in the flesh, and to hug her was to feel the strength and emotional support of all those back home.

* * *

The next morning, the sun seemed especially bright and happiness filled the house. Everyone had breakfast out by the pool and lingered there in the warmth of the morning sun. Mike had taken leave and suggested that they do some sightseeing, so they all loaded up the car and headed out about mid-morning. They began with a visit to the lovely old city of Sigtuna located northwest of Stockholm on Lake Malaren. It was founded at the beginning of the eleventh century and is Sweden's oldest town. Remnants of Viking and early-Christian heritage can be found throughout the town. John took a wheelchair along so that he could rest whenever he desired. Later in the day, they traveled to Drottningholm Palace with its French baroque gardens. The palace, which is located to the west of Stockholm, has been dubbed "The Versailles of the North." They also visited the China Pavilion, a small summerhouse at the end of the gardens, which was a birthday gift to Queen Louisa Ulrika in 1753 from her husband Adolphus Fredrick. Next stop on their tour was the Drottningholm Court Theater, the only authentic eighteenth-century stage in the world, with the original stage machinery and settings still in use. It was a wonderful, relaxing day.

That evening after dinner as they were cleaning up, Suzy turned to Joanne and asked, "How are your parents doing?"

"They're more glad than sad," she responded reflectively.

"And how about you?"

"I wish we could have the future back!"

Her answer drew understanding smiles as the message hit a deep emotional cord. It was a defining moment.

*   *   *

Keep your eyes on the future—we can learn from the past but we can't do one damn thing about it.

—Pete Keating

*   *   *

After a relaxing Saturday morning, Suzy and the Keatings drove to Skokloster Palace, one of the most splendid seventeenth-century structures in Sweden. It still retains many of the original furnishings and is noted for its collections of paintings, tapestries, arms, and armor. It houses one of the most extensive collections of old weapons in the world. John was unable to tour the palace interior because it required the negotiation of stairs, so he enjoyed the surroundings as he sat in his wheelchair in the courtyard. He felt good in the warm sun, enriched by the flow of energy that Suzy's presence had brought.

On Sunday the Keatings, with John at the helm, took Suzy on a cruise of Stockholm harbor in their boat. After departing their mooring in Djursholm, they cruised south along the western shore of Lidingo. After passing under the Stockholm-Lidingo Bridge, the sculpture garden of Carl Milles came into view high up on the bluffs of Lidingo.

"Look, Suzy," called Mike. "There is the Hand of God."

Suzy and Judy turned and looked up to where Mike was pointing.

Many of the sculptures could be seen even though they were some distance away.

"That is Mike's and my favorite," Judy explained. "It seems to have a special meaning to us now. It suggests the divine power and grace of God."

"I can imagine," replied Suzy. "It's spectacular and so significant. I love it!"

Stockholm is known for its architecture and scenic beauty and while Drottningholm Palace is known as "The Versailles of the North," the city itself has been called "Venice of the North." The view of the city from the water is breathtaking. From the harbor, they cruised out to Vaxholm and saw the fort, which guards the entrance to Vaxholm. It was a delightful day. Somehow the freedom of being on the water and seeing things from a different perspective is refreshing to the soul. The evening was spent relaxing at home.

* * *

The following morning the Keatings and Suzy sunbathed around the pool. After a leisurely lunch, Judy, Joanne, and Suzy took the Tunnelbana (Metro/subway) into the city. They strolled through Gamla Stan (Old Town) with its narrow alleys, cobblestone streets, picturesque shops, and gabled houses. The city dates from the Middle Ages, and today is home to little shops and artists' studios. They toured the Royal Treasury and walked through Kungstradgarden (Royal Garden) where they watched people playing table tennis and chess with three-foot wooden chess pieces. That evening as they sat around the dining room table, the conversation turned to what they should do tomorrow.

After some discussion, John said, "I would really like for Suzy to experience the Archipelago. Anders and Britt Gronberger have wanted us to come visit them since they are going to be out there all summer."

"Not a bad idea, John," Mike replied. "In fact, it's terrific! The last time I saw Anders he said I should bring you out when you got out of the hospital. I'll give them a call," Mike added as he rose from the table to go to the phone.

Before his retirement, Anders had been in the Air Force Section at Fo/INT and had worked closely with Mike. The two couples had become close friends. Anders and Britt had a large summerhouse on an island in the Archipelago. The first Midsummer the Keatings were in Sweden, the Gronbergers had invited the family, along with some of their Swedish friends and their families, to join them on the island for the holiday weekend. It had been a festive and memorable weekend for the four Keatings.

When Mike returned to the table he announced, "Anders was quite excited about us coming to visit. I explained about Suzy's visit from the States and your wish for her to experience the Archipelago. I told him we would bring all the food and drink. I said we would lunch on the trip out, spend the night, and then head back sometime tomorrow afternoon."

"Oh, Suzy, you are going to love it," John bubbled. "It will take us about three hours to get there through some of the most beautiful scenery you have ever seen."

*　　　*　　　*

Stockholm's celebrated Archipelago is unparalleled anywhere in the world. It extends some 40 miles out into the Baltic Sea and consists of over 24,000 islands joined together by sparkling waterways. There is a saying: "A lifetime is not long enough to discover the full beauty of the Archipelago; there is always something new to discover and be delighted by."

After breakfast, they loaded the boat with supplies and cast off on their journey into the Archipelago. The Keatings' boat was a Jurmo, a Finnish-designed inboard/outboard craft about 22-feet long with a cabin which could accommodate six to seven people comfortably inside and another four in the open deck area behind the cabin. It had a cruise speed of 15 to 20 knots. The trip through the islands was a good change-of-pace adventure from the previous days of sightseeing. As they traveled on the glistening water, the beauty of nature and the bountiful scenery enchanted them. Because of John's wish for everyone to share this experience with Suzy, they became conscious of the beauty of the moment—the aura of the present.

As they arrived at the dock, Anders and Britt came down from their house to greet them. They were especially happy to see John and were astonished by the progress he had made. They also were greatly honored that John, on his first outing since being released from the hospital, chose to visit them on their island.

Judy had brought marinated flank steaks and, while Mike grilled the steaks under the watchful eyes of Anders and John (who kept the beer flowing and the talk lively), Judy, Joanne, Suzy and Britt prepared wild rice and asparagus. This dinner was Suzy's introduction to Swedish hospitality and the traditions that go along with dinner. One could not have asked for a more charming and delightful host and hostess than Anders and Britt. She would later confess that the experience was simply overwhelming. The entire evening, set with a backdrop of tradition, hospitality, Swedish summer night, an island home, and the fresh scent of the sea, was a pleasant memory which would last a lifetime.

The next day was spent enjoying one another's company, whether exploring the island or sitting on the dock savoring the Swedish summer sun. Late in the afternoon, they bid farewell to Anders and Britt and headed back to Djursholm. Suzy had only two more days before her Saturday departure.

* * *

John wanted Suzy to see Uppsala and the hospital where he had spent the last three months, and to meet Isabelle. Uppsala is where Sweden's first university was founded in 1477. The day spent in Uppsala with Isabelle was delightful, just as the others had been. John continued to use his wheelchair frequently in order to help prevent skin ulcerations, which resulted from too much walking. His skin, much of which was burn tissue, was not tough enough to endure the demands and pressures of a prosthesis.

They visited the thirteenth-century Uppsala Cathedral, a twin-spired Gothic structure, nearly 400 feet high. They also toured the gardens of Carolus Linnaeus (1707-1778), the Swedish naturalist who was the founder of modern botany. His summer residence and the gardens are located there.

Just north of Uppsala is Gamla Uppsala (Old Uppsala). This village was the capital of the Svea kingdom around the fifth century and is the location of the Viking burial mounds from the sixth century. These mounds allegedly contain the pyres of three kings, and are considered the most important ancient monuments in Sweden.

It was a pleasant day for wandering around these sites, picnicking, and learning a little Swedish history. Suzy found Isabelle to be quietly charming and obviously very caring of John. The weather during Suzy's entire visit had been perfect. After returning home that evening, they sat around the pool relaxing and talking as time flew by unnoticed.

Friday was spent lounging around the house and pool. Actually, everyone was pretty much spent from the previous day in Uppsala and they welcomed the time to relax together. Suzy's visit had exceeded all their expectations. She had brought to John and his family all the collective feelings of confidence that they could survive this ordeal and emerge with strength, humor, and courage.

Suzy's presence had been magical. The Keatings were able, with Suzy, to process the tragedy and their concerns, to explore the future, and to reminisce about happier times. The visit had been therapeutic. They all had gained strength from their mutual bond as deeply caring friends. It was rich fertile ground upon which to build confidence for the future. Her departure was understandably difficult and tearful, but she was returning to the U.S. to validate to friends and family that the Keatings were intact. The Keatings were grateful and blessed to call Suzy Hawley a dear friend.

* * *

> *It is hard perhaps for you to see this, or if you have, I just want to reinforce what is perhaps in your own mind. But just remember...that people will love you not for what you have lost but for what you have.*
>
> *—John Davis*

* * *

Suzy Hawley
Alexandria, Virginia

July 29, 1981

Dearest Judy, Mike, John & Joanne,

What a lovely time I had with you all. I can't possibly thank you enough for providing such a warm loving spot for me. How many places could one move in for 10 days! It was a long time to have a guest—and I hope you weren't nuts by the time I left.

Returned at the proper time. However, I had, indeed, told my family that I'd be back on Sunday and wrote it on the calendar on the 26th. But I had written my itinerary with proper dates and put it on the bulletin board! The three were playing racquetball at the Pentagon when I called so I took a bus to National and called them from there. They all came to get me—explaining that they had planned to go on a big clean-up campaign Sunday in preparation for my return. The house was in remarkable shape, though, as I expected. Dave even had the boys folding the laundry, and he said that his was laid on his bed every evening…(by Mark of course.)

Called Dave Singer the minute I walked in the house. He was going to take the cuff links but Clothing Sales wasn't open on Sunday. He is a neat kid (young man!), and I'm so glad he and John are friends! He could barely contain his excitement at the prospect of seeing John.

Have tried and tried to reach Pat but without success. I've called at all sorts of odd times. He may be on vacation—or out in San Diego house hunting. He knew when I'd be returning so I'll wait for his call.

Called Sandra and she was a delight. She sounds like a dear sister and friend—and was so eager for news of John's recovery and of life in the Keating household. You'll be **thrilled** *to know I finally sent the tray!*

Called Mr. Mullin and we had a long and enthusiastic discussion. As you can imagine he was delighted at John's progress. I am sure he thinks the power of Episcopal prayer had much to do with it. And, even though I tweaked him on it, I must agree with him. I also spoke with Cannon Martin—and he, as does everyone, thinks you all are wonderful—and certainly come from "strong stock!"

I spoke with both Mrs. Sundt and Mrs. Staples. They were very appreciative of your desire to let them know how things were going. I called Susy Cromwell—after Dave gave me her number. She's away for the summer, but her mother and I had a nice chat and she'll get the word to Susy that the letter was thoroughly enjoyed! Haven't been able to get Bowden's number. Dave H. will try to get it today or I'll drop her a note to call me.

Sent you all a gift to celebrate John's birth and the most recent gift of his life. You all gave me the idea when looking for the sailboat. I have admired the sailboats I sent you for well over a year. It gives me such a thrill to send them to my beloved friends. It further connects the families in my heart because I always remember the two silver sailboats that Mummy had on a circular mirror on our dining table when I was very young. And, of course, they carry the significance of the wind being back in the Keating sails.

You did such a super human job of "doing Sweden" with me and the experience was marvelous. What an incredible way to see Stockholm and its environs!—Judy, I couldn't believe it! Still more gifts as I open my bag. Thank you for the rooster.

Must go and fool in my garden and prepare the windows for the "great work." I adore you all and hope you know I am available as "listener" for anyone of the four special Keatings who would like to write.

Love,
Suzy

* * *

St. Albans School
Mount St. Alban
Washington, D.C.

Headmaster's Study

July 31, 1981

Dear John:

I was in Massachusetts for a week, and what a delight it was to get back to school and receive a call from Mrs. Hawley. Her good news about seeing you and the improvement you have made was just what I wanted to hear! Then your letter came, and I am doubly pleased to have heard from you. It is great to hear that you walked out of the hospital, and even greater to learn that you are able to play Frisbee! Be careful though. Don't forget what happened to your classmate in the Bishop's garden!

The summer programs are winding down at St. Albans and the place will be quiet for a few weeks; but football camp gets underway on the 20th. I am afraid it is going to be a fairly small and inexperienced team this year, but they appear to have a lot of spirit.

I know you are looking forward to seeing Dave and William. It is great that they will get to Sweden. Do keep in touch, I wish you all the best. Thanks for the good news that lifted my spirits so much.

Sincerely yours,

Mark H. Mullin
Headmaster

*　　　*　　　*

Chapter Six

Dave, Billy, and Tom
(August–September, 1981)

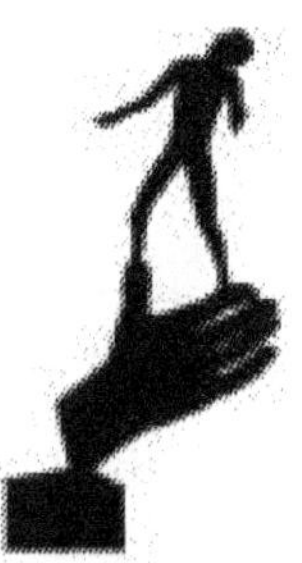

*　　　*　　　*

Let people help you—I don't mean the hospital staff, but folks with which you later come in contact; you will be surprised at how many folks really do want to help and how many fine people there are in the outside world.

—*Burr Piggot*

*　　　*　　　*

The next two weeks were spent savoring the memories of Suzy's visit and anticipating the arrival of Dave Singer and Billy Mondale, two of John's classmates from St. Albans. They were scheduled to arrive sometime Sunday afternoon, the 9th of August. The exact time was not known as the two youngsters were traveling with Eurailpasses.

Isabelle was visiting for the weekend, and the Keating family decided to spend the morning on the boat out in the Archipelago. They departed around 9:30 and had been cruising for about an hour with John at the helm while the others sunbathed. John had taken his prosthesis off and was standing on his good leg leaning against the raised helmsman's chair when the wake of a passing boat caused their boat to roll unexpectedly. John had not anticipated the sudden roll and lost his balance. He instinctively put his injured leg out to regain his balance but because he did not have his prosthesis on, he fell, jamming the stump of his leg on a cushioned bench.

The bandage on John's leg immediately became saturated with blood, so the boat excursion was aborted and they turned for home. The Keatings moored their boat in front of their house but used a public dock about a half mile north for embarking and disembarking passengers. As they passed their mooring and proceeded north to the dock, Mike noticed two young men sitting on their front porch enjoying the sun and the view. (Dave Singer had visited the Keatings the Christmas of 1979, so he was familiar with Stockholm and the house.)

"Look," Mike exclaimed. "That must be Dave and Billy."

"You're right," said Judy as she waved to them.

John was below with Isabelle but sat up and attempted to peer out the side window. John's parents and Joanne waved to the two, and they returned the wave, but the Keatings were not sure Dave and Billy recognized who they were or noticed the Stars and Stripes being flown from the boat's stern. They proceeded to the dock where everyone disembarked. Earlier in the day, they had driven down to the dock and fortunately had John's wheelchair in the trunk of the car so it was fairly easy to move John to the car and return home. Mike returned the boat to its mooring and paddled to shore in a small rubber dingy.

Meanwhile, Judy, Joanne, Isabelle, and John drove back to the house. John was quite excited in anticipation of seeing Dave and Billy again. When they arrived, Judy wheeled John around by the pool where Dave and Billy were relaxing.

"Hey!" John yelled.

Dave and Billy looked up and jumped to their feet. "Johnny," Dave yelled. "How ya doin'?"

John, Dave, and Billy were all talking at once; but nonetheless, there was communication amongst the simultaneous talking. Their greetings and welcome were genuine and emotional. It was very much like Suzy's reaction two weeks before. Dave and Billy were here hugging John and they felt a tremendous sense of relief. Their friend was alive, and they were finally with him.

"Hey, guys," John's mother interrupted, "John needs to have his leg looked after. He fell while we were out on the boat."

"Yeah, I did. Hey, you guys! Isabelle, this is Dave Singer and Billy Mondale. Dave and Billy, this is Isabelle Pettersson."

This break in the action permitted John's parents and Joanne to welcome the boys and give them hugs.

"Mom," Dave said as he hugged Judy.

"Welcome to Sweden, and thank you for coming," Judy said. "You can't imagine how much this means to all of us."

"We're glad we had the opportunity to come, and thank you for inviting us," Billy replied.

"We need to get John inside so Isabelle can have a look at his leg," Mike insisted. "I'll wheel him into his room and Isabelle can attend to him."

"Can we come and talk to him while…" Dave asked.

"Of course," Mike interrupted. "Come on."

They proceeded to John's room where he moved himself from the wheelchair onto his bed. Mike and Judy adjourned to the living room while Isabelle began unwrapping the bloody dressing. No sooner had the two sat down than Dave and Billy smartly entered the room. "I think we'll join you all since we're not quite up to seeing what is underneath that bandage," Dave confessed. "It's one thing to imagine the horror of an amputation; it's quite another to see it. We're just not up to it."

"Don't apologize," Mike said. "Initially, I even found the word *amputation* difficult to say, and I still get uneasy when the doctor refers to John's stump!"

They talked about how the two boys' families were doing, what they had been doing this summer, and how college life was at Yale and Brown.

Isabelle interrupted them, announcing: "John's fine. There is no damage and I've redressed his leg. He's putting on his prosthesis and will be out in a minute."

There were two sighs of relief. First, it was great that he had not injured himself when he fell, and second, that Isabelle was astute enough not to go into any details. Then, when John walked into the room, their faces lit up with the joy of seeing John on his feet and walking.

Everyone gathered around the pool where they enjoyed a leisurely lunch with the boys talking mostly about their friends in Washington, highlighted with gossip. About mid-afternoon, Isabelle had to return to Uppsala but agreed to meet them again on Thursday after John's appointment with Dr. Hakelius.

*　　　*　　　*

Now I know why your country is so great!

—Tom Yamasaki

*　　　*　　　*

Monday, August 10th, was John's twentieth birthday. The day was spent preparing for the celebration that was to be an evening dinner party around the pool. Dave and Billy were a great help to Joanne and Judy as they set up tables and chairs around the pool, accompanied Judy to the grocery store, and assisted in the food preparation. Mike had gone to the Embassy, but had promised to return home early in the afternoon to help. John, Dave, and Billy were able to keep a running conversation going amongst all the activity. It was a busy day.

In order to provide Dave and Billy an opportunity to get acquainted with some of the guests, John's mother had arranged the seating so there would be three tables of four. John, Dave, and Billy would each host a table containing another male and two females. As anticipated, the three boys kept the activity at their tables active and lively. The guests included American, British, Swedish, and Finnish youngsters. At John's table were Dave Moss, Beth Thomson, and Vivete Olson; Dave hosted Bobby Thomson, Caroline Puntan, and Helena Hokanson; and Billy hosted Tim Puntan, Asa Thoden, and Joanne.

The evening was picture perfect. The sky was clear, weather warm, and the beautiful sunset lasted a couple of hours. It was well into the night before it became completely dark. The kids had a great time celebrating with John not only his twentieth birthday but also his survival of having taken 16,000 volts. It was a very special occasion, particularly for Tim and Caroline who had witnessed the accident.

* * *

You'll find that it is truly the simple things in life, and the relationships you make that make life worthwhile.

—*Teddy Kennedy*

* * *

The boys slept late the next morning, and, when they did awake, they were ready for a morning dip. The water in the pool was heated but quite refreshing.

"Billy," Dave said. "We've got to take a swim in the Baltic. We've come all this way, and we've got to be able to say we did it!"

"Let's do it!" Billy responded.

The two headed around the side of the house and down the front lawn. John moved to the front porch from where he could observe them. If the pool water was refreshing at 75 degrees, the Baltic was eye opening at 62 degrees. While their bodies might have been numb from the night before, they were awake now. They romped around for a short while and then concluded that it might be prudent to call it quits. The Keatings had a sauna, which had been turned on in anticipation of its need, and Dave and Billy were grateful. When they had thawed out, the boys decided they would go sightseeing in Stockholm. Judy drove them to the subway, and the three were on their way.

Their first stop was to visit the Royal Flagship Wasa, a seventeenth-century man-of-war ordered built by Gustavus Adolphus II. Unfortunately, the king did not listen to his naval engineers and insisted his own design ideas be incorporated. He continually advised them during its construction, changing requirements, and adding features. The engineers knew the ship was becoming more and more unstable, but their arguments failed to persuade the king. Finally, on a bright, sunny Sunday, August 10th, 1628, the ship set sail on her maiden voyage. Not far from the dock a gust of wind caused the ship to keel over, and she sank into the murky waters of Stockholm harbor. Attempts to salvage were made but none were successful. However, more than 50 of her bronze cannons were saved.

It was not until 300 years later that Anders Franzen, an amateur marine archaeologist, discovered the ship. Allegedly, he plotted the reported location of ships that lost anchors by having them snagged by something on the harbor's bottom. The concentration of these reports, when plotted on a chart of the harbor, led Franzen to the *Wasa*. To his credit and subsequent fame, he undertook one of the most amazing salvaging projects of the century when, under his direction, the *Wasa* was lifted from the bottom, some 110 feet below, and towed to shallower water. On April 24th, 1961, amidst great fanfare and press coverage, the *Wasa* was raised. She had lain on the bottom for three centuries, and to everyone's delight she was unbelievably well preserved. The artifacts were plentiful and dramatically illustrated the royal tastes of that time. Today, the *Wasa* is housed in a specially constructed museum that is kept extremely humid. The story of the restoration of the ship and its preservation is remarkable. The ship is considered the world's oldest identified ship and has become a major tourist attraction.

The boys dropped by the Sheridan Hotel for lunch. John had worked there the previous summer as a waiter.

"I used to work those tables over there," John said pointing to a group of tables across the room. "It was really funny. I received numerous compliments, especially from English-speaking patrons, on how good my English was."

John paused, and then added, "You know, I never had the heart to tell them I was an American. I figured it was better for them to think I was Swedish. They were so nice and considerate, not condescending at all. I guess I wanted them to go home with a very positive impression of Sweden and the Swedish people."

"Oh!" John continued. "One time, this guy was sitting with his family and told me I spoke almost perfect English. Imagine that 'almost perfect English.' Wouldn't the faculty at St. Albans be impressed?"

They all laughed. But they also understood John's position and his desire to project Sweden in a most favorable light.

After lunch they took a boat ride and ended up at the Royal Palace. It was here that John's prosthesis suffered metal fatigue and gave way. John fell to the ground, but fortunately they were on gravel at the time. He was not injured, but his leg was bent almost 90 degrees outward and gave the appearance of a horrible fracture. Billy decided that it might help if he tried to straighten it, so he grabbed John's foot and began attempting to straighten it. Dave was holding the upper part of the leg so Billy could get some leverage. The temptation was too much for John to just sit there like nothing was going on. As passersby were stopping to see what had happened, he let out a bone-chilling scream, so loud that it startled Dave and Billy—and everyone else for that matter. The three began laughing as the passersby decided it was some kind of staged prank and John was not at all hurt or in pain. The Palace guard, who had moved towards them when John fell, thinking he was hurt, stepped back to his post and regained his stoic pose.

The three made a comical sight trying to get John down the hill to the sidewalk. First of all, he could not put any weight on his broken prosthesis, which was grotesquely bent outward to the left. John had his right arm around Billy's neck so Billy could support him and John could stand on his right leg. But Dave could offer no support with his shoulder because John did not have a left arm. Dave ended up pushing John's left side and trying to support him by grabbing his belt whenever John hopped on his good leg. Eventually, they made it to a pay phone where Dave dialed the Keatings' home.

"No answer. Mom must be out," John concluded. "I'll try Dad at the Embassy."

"Defense Attaché Office," Sandy said.

"Sandy, this is John. Is my Dad there?"

"Sure, just a minute."

There was a short pause.

"John, what's up?"

"We are down at the Palace and one of the metal bars on my leg broke and the other is badly bent. I'm essentially immobile. Called Mom, but she's not home. Could you come get us?"

"Tord has my car at the moment and is out on an errand. Let me check to see where the other three vehicles are."

There was another short pause.

"John, we don't have any vehicles available right now. Just grab a taxi and come on over to the Embassy. You can catch a ride home with me."

"Okay. See you shortly."

* * *

And don't forget you're a "strapper." (Strapping, virile, young man, who's a ladies man.)

—Ellen Singer

* * *

The following day, John was essentially confined to a wheelchair. One can only hop so much. The boys spent the morning hanging around the pool, and in the afternoon everyone went out on the boat to view Stockholm from the water. They cruised for the better part of four hours with the boys checking out the topless sunbathing beauties along the island shores.

The next morning, Judy drove the boys and Joanne to Uppsala where John had an appointment with Dr. Hakelius. She and John also dropped by the Go Skolen with John's broken prosthesis.

Robert and Lennart, the two technicians at the Go Skolen, stared in absolute disbelief as John entered their workshop in his wheelchair with his bent and broken leg in his lap. "The American" had done the impossible, for this was, after all, Swedish steel and not subject to failure at the hands of mere mortals. They could not believe what they saw. It was a mystery. They had never seen anything like it before. They joked with John as they worked on repairing the prosthesis by welding two braces on either side of the leg. The braces added significant weight to the leg, but it was repaired, and John was able to walk out of the Go Skolen.

While John and his mother were at the Go Skolen and Dr. Hakelius' office, Joanne, Dave, and Billy did some sightseeing. Eventually, they all rendezvoused, including Isabelle, and picnicked in the park before heading back to Djursholm.

Saturday, Dave and Billy were scheduled to depart, so the boys spent Friday together, talking and planning for the future.

"You have got to visit me at Yale, Johnny, when you get back," Dave said. "When will you be leaving? Do you know?"

"It should be September a year," John replied. "And I'll definitely stop by for a weekend. We probably will go up to Maine to visit relatives, and then I know Dad has to debrief in Washington. I could fly down from Maine for a weekend, and my folks could pick me up when they come through New Haven on their way to D.C."

"Let's plan on it then."

Saturday came and, of course, was difficult. The visit had been too short, but Dave and Billy left feeling very exuberant because they were going home to tell Washington that John had not changed one single, solitary bit. John Keating was doing great! And they anticipated the joy of spreading the word.

*　　　*　　　*

> *Keep up the great progress, all of you. The nice thing about being part of a super family is we can share our triumphs and travails alike!*
>
> —*Pete Keating*

*　　　*　　　*

On Monday, Judy returned to work part-time. She had been employed in the Embassy by the Consular Section as Consular Investigation Assistance since April 1980, but had taken a leave of absence after John's accident. This employment was in addition to her major responsibilities as the wife of the Defense Attaché. Because of the requirement for John to be followed closely by the doctors in Uppsala, she could only work three days a week, but Bob Dorr, the American Consul, was happy to have her back.

While the representational duties were demanding, the Keatings managed to cope, and since July had been able to keep up with their commitments. One of these events was the Mini-Baltic sailboat race hosted by the Swedish Air Force Wing at Tullinge just outside of Stockholm. It pitted several crews from the Wing against an equal number of two-man crews from the American Embassy. After the race, the teams adjourned to the sauna, drank beer, and enjoyed one another's company. This was followed by a dinner and party games. It was a delightful afternoon and evening, made especially memorable because the Wing Commander, Colonel Bernt Osth, had specifically invited John to attend. John rode on the Committee Boat and was able to join in the activities and camaraderie.

Two weeks after Dave and Billy departed, Tom Liddy arrived and spent a week with the Keatings. Tom graduated from St. Albans a year after John, but they had been on the swimming team together and had become good friends. Tom was traveling in India and Egypt and took the opportunity to swing by Stockholm on the way home. Tom was a delightful houseguest and the entire family enjoyed his company. John, Joanne, and Tom played Frisbee and did some sightseeing. Although it was now September and the weather was becoming a little cooler, they still enjoyed being outdoors and going out on the boat. One evening, Carita and Olof Thoden, the Finnish Defense Attaché and their two daughters, Asa and Lena, came to dinner. It was a delightful evening and these two young Finnish beauties smote Tom, like Dave and Billy before him. It was a great visit, just like Dave and Billy's, and Tom left with the knowledge and reassurance that John was all right and still a Freebird.

* * *

I just wanted you to know that I can relate to what you're going through. It can be such a bitch at first but you can't let it slow you down.

—Jeff Ingraham

* * *

Dr. Hakelius was pleased with John's progress as he examined his leg and the healing of the stump.

"All the wounds have healed and look good," he reported. "The skin is very thin over the stump though."

"What does that mean?" asked John.

"Well, John, the tissue covering the stump is scar tissue from the burns and consequently is very thin," he explained. "Hopefully this skin will toughen up enough to support a prosthesis. We'll just have to wait and see. Later on we might attempt to graft some skin onto the stump if need be. In a worse case, you might have problems with wearing a prosthesis full time, especially at first, but with time everything should work out."

John related to the doctor that he had been playing Frisbee, doing a lot of sightseeing, and had had another friend from Washington visit for a week. Dr. Hakelius was pleased that John was active and told him that he hoped they could fit him with a new prosthesis in the near future that would enable him to use his own knee.

"And I understand you are still seeing quite a bit of Isabelle," Hakelius stated.

"Yes, sir. Sure am."

* * *

We are convinced that John has some special inner strength and an enormous reservoir of whatever is required to look adversity in the eye and come away laughing.

—Dan Singer

* * *

One of the things John wished to accomplish but had been unable to do because of all the company from the U.S., was to pay a return call on the British Ambassador. The Ambassador's visit to Uppsala had been very meaningful to John and he wished to walk into the Ambassador's office and say, "Thanks!"

"Ambassador Murray's Office."

"Hello, this is Colonel Keating. I'm the American Defense Attaché and would like to make an appointment for my son John to pay a courtesy call on the Ambassador."

"Ah, yes, Colonel Keating. Your son was the one injured at Storlien several months ago. Wing Commander Barcilon has been keeping us abreast of his progress. How is he doing?"

"He's doing fine, thank you. He has been released from the hospital and is home now. He would very much like to make a short call on the Ambassador and thank him for coming to visit him in Uppsala."

"The Ambassador's schedule is completely filled through the remainder of the week," she paused. "But, let's see. What time tomorrow would be most convenient for you?"

"I thought you said his schedule was full."

"It is, but the Ambassador will make the time to see John. Would two o'clock be all right?"

"That will be fine."

"Will you be coming also?"

"No. I think this is just between John and the Ambassador."

"Fine. We'll be expecting John at two o'clock tomorrow. The Ambassador will be very pleased to see John up and about."

*　　　*　　　*

We only get as far as we strive to get—no one else can do it for us nor give it to us.

—Barbara Leiser

*　　　*　　　*

Dave Singer
Yale University
New Haven, Connecticut

September 7, 1981

Keating Family,

Well, I'm at school now. I got home and immediately found out that I had four days in D.C. before I had to go away to soccer camp. The Yale coach got me a job at a camp, where I taught soccer for a couple of hours a day and worked out the rest of the time. Consequently, I'm in great shape; I'm also playing well. Looks as if I'll get some playing time. Classes have just begun and I've almost got my schedule set. At Yale you get two weeks to shop around for courses until we have to turn in our schedules. It's a nice luxury this way; theoretically, you never get a bad professor (?).

We made it to Brussels all right, and our flight only left four hours late. We made our connection from JFK to National, no problem.

Steph got a letter from John and informed me that he/you is/are taking Swedish. I would like you, John, to send me a course listing for the

Spring from Stockholm University. Actually, I really don't need it but if I get one then I know you must have gone down and found out about courses. Next—send me a copy of your registration form for the Spring. (Take English—it'll be an easy A over there.)

I've just been out-stereod—someone across the quad has a huge stereo and is blasting it out their window. I conceded and turned mine off. I figure I'm better off anyway—he has to change the records.

Steph is doing real well. She was confused and lonesome the first couple of days but once registration and everything got underway, the blues left and its been clear sailing ever since. She is taking some pretty tough courses, which unfortunately means she will not have time to do my homework. I guess it won't get done.

I haven't had much time to enjoy "college life" as it were, because of soccer (we have two practices a day on weekends), but it is probably better for my digestive system and my brain—not to mention classes and soccer.

After a traumatic experience in High School with Spanish, I've decided to try it again. I'm also taking two history courses, one on Europe starting at WW I and one on the colonies. And an economics course for good measure.

Joanne—By now you must be settled into school. I'd be interested to hear about whether or not teaching will be your occupation this spring again.

Mom—Remember be careful who you give visas to.

Steph is trying to find time to come over to Sweden. I think she is checking into Spring-Summer. Mom and Dad are doing well. I think they're in Europe now, but I'm not sure. Did Tom show up?

Johnny—Say hi to Isabelle for me.

I feel like going into an elaborate "thank you" for having William and me, but I think the family knows how much I enjoy being with them and

I hope my thanks is conveyed in a different manner. I hope I have many more opportunities to spend time with you all.

See ya soon.

Love,
Starsky

* * *

Michael Keating
University of Wisconsin
Madison, Wisconsin

September 17, 1981

Dear John,

Hi! Probably thought I died or something, but I'm actually alive and well in Madison. I got back and went to work, which was much easier than I thought it would be to take. I came down to school in my "new" seventy-five dollar Mercury Montigo ('68). It's a real beaut.

I've spent more time in the library in three weeks of school than I did my first two years. I don't know what's gotten into me. I'm still recuperating from the Wis. upset over Mich. who are #1 ranked (Wis. is real low) last weekend. School is cool; I've got two political courses, literature, and Spanish. I expect at least one "A" and no "C's." (I've never seen any of my family pass out (except John a couple of times).)

I'm living close to campus in a three-room downstairs flat which is one of four apts. I still can't believe Madtown. Wow! 42,000 students and more than half female. I'm really not doing much besides housekeeping (it needs lots of work), schooling, and otherwise.

I saw my bro Jim this summer. He's cool. I met his girlfriend and she's a cutie. We all went to the Mole Lake bluegrass fest and had a **great** *time. John's out in California and I saw Peg (his bride to be even though he doesn't know it) before she flew out there to be with him (and work). She's a nice girl and my Mom likes her.*

How'd the summer end up? I'm sure you kept busy with your friends etc. Hi to all and a lotta love to anyone else that you see that I know.

Hasta luego!

Michael

* * *

Nichola Barcilon
London, England

September 22, 1981

Dear John,

Time goes by and I thought it was time to drop you a line or two just to make sure you're not feeling forgotten.

I always hear about you from my parents and in case you're beginning to think I'm too clever that's whom I got your address from. I hope you don't mind this occasional writing of mine!

Over here I continue to work very hard (writing most of the time for my own pleasure) at my opticians in the heart of London and enjoying the good things in life. My car, which is a mini and also a sore talking point at the moment (Please don't say anything about this to my parents. No point in worrying them.), is still on the road but has got a beautiful dent in the rear due to another woman's careless driving. Don't say typical! I am about to go into battle with the insurance companies to get it all repaired and paid for.

As you know my parents are due home in a few weeks time, which of course I'm looking forward to. I hope that when you have to return to America it would be possible for you to stop over with us in England that way of course I could see "Animal" and friend (you) again to make up for not seeing you a second time in Sweden.

Keep fighting the things you have to fight and keep looking ahead not back. I think of you and admire you a lot and wish that I had some of the power you have.

Take care, have more and more fun.

Love,
Nichola

* * *

Thomas P. Liddy
Fort Washington, Maryland

September 28, 1981

Hey John,

I bet that you are speaking some serious Swedish by now. I am finally back in the groove here in Washington. For about a week I was just not at all back in the States yet. It's nice to be back though.

I just can't tell you what a really good time I had in Stockholm. It was a hell of a way to end my trip. Tell your Mom and Dad how grateful I am.

Now that I've gotten that out of the way, I've got to tell you that I just bought a car. It's a deep blue, 19 hundred and 72 MALIBU. She really runs well. I've got to put a new stereo in her though.

The more I think about it the more I'm convinced that you've just got to spend a few days with me when you get back here. I went to a Commodore's Concert at the Capitol Center last week.

I haven't heard from Dave since I've come back. I don't have his new address at Yale; so when you write him, tell him to send me something in the mail.

When I get those pictures developed, I'll send them to you. I'll send you some other crap too, including that book I owe you. I really haven't gotten my stuff together yet! To tell you the truth I don't think I ever will completely.

Take care of yourself,

Tom

* * *

Chapter Seven

Returning to Normal (October 1981–September 1982)

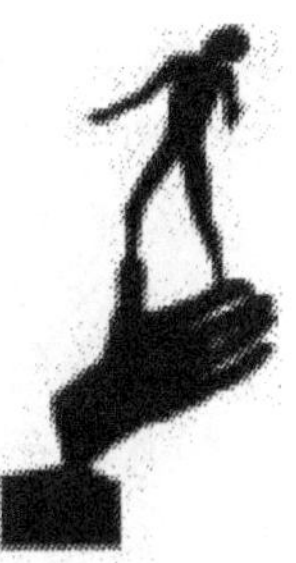

*　　　*　　　*

Soon you folks will be on your last year in Sweden. I do hope you have less trouble. How lucky we don't know what is ahead.

—*Great Grandma Burgess*

*　　　*　　　*

With the coming of autumn, the pace of activity began to increase. Joanne's godfather, Phil Johnson, passed through Stockholm for a short visit early in October. The Keatings hosted a dinner party for twenty-one, honoring the Barcilons, the first Friday in October. The Barcilons were completing their tour and returning to England. The following evening, Jacquie and Judy attended the ballet and saw Rudolf Nureyev dance. Bob had told Jacquie that he was not interested so Jacquie had invited Judy. Since the girls were out to a cultural event, Mike invited Bob over to the house to watch a "cultural" movie with John, Joanne, and himself. The movie: "Smokey and the Bandit;" the refreshments: beer and popcorn.

Mid-October brought a visit by Secretary of Defense Caspar Weinberger, his wife, and party. The SECDEF's five-day visit was hectic for Judy and Mike, but enjoyable, and the Swedes' gracious hospitality demonstrated their efficiency and concern for detail. The Weinberger visit was closely followed by a two-day visit by Brigadier General Don Goodman, the Assistant Vice Director for Attachés and Training, Defense Intelligence Agency. He no sooner departed when Mike learned of the untimely visit of a Soviet submarine which had run aground in the territorial waters near the Swedish naval base of Karlskrona. October had been a busy month for the Defense Attaché Office in Stockholm.

In November, the Keatings traveled to Germany where Mike had meetings with military officials in Stuttgart and Ramstein. John was now using his new prosthesis, which permitted him to bend his knee while walking. Although he walked with a slight limp and continued to have problems with skin ulcerations, he felt he had come a long way since the accident. The medical personnel at Wiesbaden, who examined him, were very complimentary of the medical care he had received and impressed by his positive attitude.

December brought a visit from Kent Penfield, one of John's fraternity brothers from the University of New Hampshire. Then came the Christmas holidays and the beginning of a new year. It had been an eventful year, summarized by the Keatings' Holiday letter.

*　　　*　　　*

The Keatings
American Embassy
Stockholm, Sweden

January 1982

Happy New Year—

Nineteen eighty-one was an eventful year in Sweden—visitors ranged from Sec. Def. Weinberger to a Soviet submarine. It kept us very busy with official representational functions and our jobs at the Embassy. Mike continues to find being Defense and Air Attaché most interesting and Judy finds working in the Consular Section (in Swedish) balances the social schedule.

Joanne attends the International School where she helps the teachers with the lower grade students and works privately part-time improving her reading skills. She enjoys her days and is speaking some Swedish.

John had a rough year beginning with an auto accident in Washington, D.C., a year ago Thanksgiving. He was a passenger but sustained injuries to the neck and arm, which hospitalized him and caused him to miss his final exams at UNH. Second semester found him trying to "make-up" and stay with the program. This didn't work out and he returned to Sweden to "sort it all out."

While the entire family was on a ski trip in Northern Sweden, John accidentally came in contact with 16,000 volts of electricity. He had climbed a railroad tank car in a rail yard nearby—unaware of the "hot" overhead wire. Emergency travel had him at the burn unit in Uppsala within eight hours, via helicopter and airplane. The excellent care he received and his own strength combined to save his life, but it was necessary to amputate his left arm at the shoulder and left leg at mid-calf. Many operations and 98 days later he walked out of the hospital 40 pounds lighter.

His recovery since July has been remarkable and he has regained weight, strength, and mastered walking, dancing, Frisbee throwing, Swedish, and even played squash. His sense of humor and courage helped all of us to cope with the situation.

Fantastic support from many friends and relatives carried us through the hardest period. A series of five young men visited from the U.S. to check on John and found him "A-okay". We appreciate all the cards, letters, calls, and prayers and will continue to draw strength from them.

We return to the U.S. in mid-September 1982 with plans for John and Joanne to continue their education. Judy hopes to finally use her master's degree in counseling on a professional level. Mike is waiting to hear what his next assignment will be.

We're ready to return but will certainly leave many good friends behind in Sweden.

Mike & Judy

* * *

Not all of the Keatings' friends learned of the accident in a timely manner. Those living in the Washington area were initially alerted and then kept abreast of John's progress through a very efficient grapevine. Generally, military friends around the world also were informed through common friends and contemporaries. However, some civilian friends, who were not on the grapevine circuit, were quite shocked to receive the Christmas letter. One such individual was Peter Armstrong, one of Mike's childhood friends who was an Assistant Dean at Dartmouth College. Pete and Mike had been friends since the early '50s when their fathers were stationed together at the Army War College at Carlisle Barracks, Pennsylvania. Pete wrote immediately upon hearing the news.

* * *

Peter Hoyle Armstrong
Dartmouth College
Hanover, New Hampshire

February 16, 1982

Dear Mike and Judy,

With disbelief and shock I read your News of 1981 after work today and am writing immediately to share with you my very belated thoughts and prayers for John as he continues his remarkable recovery. He indeed must be an exceptional young man to be able to face his new life with such courage and at the same time bring the comfort you speak of to those closest to him. While my heart truly aches for each of you, I am so proud to know that a senseless tragedy can unearth such inner power in someone so young—to positively go forward to face and conquer these unpredictable obstacles in his life.

You have every right to be so proud of both John and Joanne and, as their parents, ***this*** *friend is so very proud of* ***you****.*

May this New Year bring each of you much needed happiness and sunshine. I shall also be more than eager to hear where you will be next stationed. How I wish this might be somewhere in New England next October!

My special love to the four of you,

Peter

P.S. I have written this note in great haste—to be mailed tomorrow; thus my thoughts may not be adequately expressed on paper, but you will certainly understand the feelings I've tried to extend to you.

*　　*　　*

On January 7th, John returned to the hospital in Uppsala for his sixth operation. The operation consisted of skin grafting. He remained hospitalized for 14 days after which he returned home and began a series of visits back to the Go Skolen to be fitted for and learn to use a smaller, lighter prosthesis. It was not long before he was walking almost naturally. However, he did experience the skin "breaking down" resulting in ulcerated areas on the stump. He encountered and tolerated the normal frustrations associated with such delays because he recognized it simply takes time for these types of wounds to heal.

John began studying Swedish in a free course along with several immigrants. He enjoyed the course and the people he met. In addition, he began working at the Embassy commissary. He assisted Dave Kushner, the commissary officer, in attending the store. It was a good activity for John, permitting him to meet many of the Embassy personnel who had sent their good wishes and prayers for his recovery. Gradually, the gloom of the long winter faded and the spring flowers began to dot the landscape in a beautiful mural of color and rebirth.

Anders Julin invited John to lunch at the Kallaren Aurora, a famous restaurant in Gamla Stan. Anders had received two tapes, which his stepfather in England had promised to send, and wanted to personally present them to John. During lunch, the owner of the restaurant and Olaf Palme, the former Prime Minister, stopped by the table to greet Anders, whom they both knew. It was quite an honor for John to meet them.

The more than five hours of tapes were an excellent source of information and insight into the world of the handicapped. Not only did John gain useful, practical information about daily living, but he also learned a little about philosophy and the seeming ignorance and indifference of bureaucracies. Most of all, Anders' stepfather encouraged John to live his life to the fullest.

"You have had extremely bad luck in having had the accident; but good luck in having survived it," he remarked.

He encouraged John to take good care of himself and commented on the fact that in his experience approximately half of those who suffer a tragedy get on with their lives, while the other half whither in self-pity.

He said that moving on requires three things, "Attitude, attitude, and attitude."

He quoted Act III of Shakespeare's *Twelfth Night*: "In nature there's no blemish but the mind; None can be called deformed but the unkind."

One thought which capsulated his wealth of information was his observation: "John, people will accept a man with one arm, but they will not accept a man with a plastic hand."

* * *

This was the last summer for the Keatings in Sweden, and they made several boat trips into the Archipelago visiting Swedish friends. They also visited Erik and Karen Hammarskjold and their two children, Maria and Niklas, on the island of Gotland. Erik was the nephew of Dag Hammarskjold, the United Nations Secretary-General from 1953 until his death in a plane crash in 1961.

The Keatings drove south to Nynashamn where they took the car ferry to Visby, a trip of about five hours. Karen's parents had a summer stuga on the island and the three-day visit there was delightful and fun filled. Erik and Karen were gracious hosts and served as tour guides as the two families explored the island's cliffs, old rock formations, beaches, and rolling countryside dotted with colorful poppies.

They picnicked among the ruins from the Middle Ages and walked the beaches, collecting small stones and shells. The city of Visby and the island of Gotland, with all of its medieval charm, was a fascinating place to visit and relax with dear friends.

Three weeks later, the Keatings traveled to Finland to visit the Pihlajas and Thodens. Kalevi Pihlaja, a Professor of Chemistry at the University of Turku, is a relative of Judy's and had visited the Lane family in Maine a few years earlier. Kalevi's grandmother, Hannah, and Judy's grandmother, Jenny, were sisters. Kalevi met the Keatings upon their arrival in Turku and spent the day showing them the city. That evening the Keatings had dinner with Kalevi, his wife, Tytti, and their three girls, Leila-Marja, Paivi-Leena, and Riita-Liisa.

During coffee following a delicious dinner, Kalevi turned to John and asked, "What would you really like to do while here in Finland?"

"We're unfortunately limited by time because we're driving to Helsinki tomorrow to visit friends, but if I had the time, I would like to drive to the border and look across into Russia. Just to say I've seen it," John answered.

"Well," Kalevi began, "that is a beautiful trip. You would certainly enjoy it, as you would travel through very scenic countryside. But remember, when you look across the border, you are not looking into Russia!"

His expression accentuated the fact that Finland has not forgotten that the land in question was seized by Russia in 1939 after Russia attacked Finland in violation of a nonaggression agreement between the two countries.

The next day, the Keatings drove to Helsinki and enjoyed the sightseeing and shopping. They had been invited by Olof and Carita Thoden to visit them at their stuga, which was about an hour's drive from Helsinki on the Gulf of Finland. It was a most enjoyable time of hiking in the forest, relaxing in the sauna between dips into the cold waters of the Gulf, and savoring herring cooked over an open fire on the beach during the several hours of twilight.

The summer passed quickly, and as the days grew shorter and the weather colder, the Keatings began to prepare to depart.

* * *

You learn a lot about people but more importantly, you learn **a lot** *about yourself. That in itself is rewarding. I consider myself a*

strong individual; from what I've heard about you and the way you are, I think you will come out of this a stronger person yourself.
—Jeff Ingraham

* * *

John continued to receive letters from family and friends during this period of time. They were informative, occasionally funny, and reflective of the trials and travails of college, family, romance, and adjustments. They were indeed music for the soul for John as he regained his strength, began socializing again, and worked part-time.

Bitsy Cronin sent news of her experiences working at a camp during the summer of 1981 and of her studies at the University of Alabama. She related how she missed Washington and all the wonderful mutual friends they had there. She called over the Christmas holidays, which gave John a major boost. Bitsy's mother, Mary Cronin, wrote often with news of Bitsy, Bitsy's grandmother and aunt, and the family dog Liz.

Susy Cromwell was a prolific letter writer and an articulate correspondent. Over the span of time that she wrote, her maturity was evident as she shared her insightful thoughts freely. Her activities included hiking, traveling, time with her family, studies at Princeton, acting, music, and camping. Her stories of her times while at Squam Lake in New Hampshire, both in the summer and winter, were humorous and entertaining. "A bunch of modern day Waltons, we are," she concluded.

Tom Liddy forwarded news of the New York Yankees and the crash of an Air Florida jet into the 14th Street Bridge. He also wrote of John's return to the States adding, "Everybody is looking forward to your return. I keep telling everyone that you and I talked about them a lot. So play it up when you get home."

Stephanie Singer was an amazingly entertaining letter writer. Her enthusiasm was evident in her descriptions of places and people. Life for Steph was a smorgasbord to be enjoyed to the fullest. Her uplifting letters were always anticipated and enjoyed. "Oh, and my Mom bought me sheets and a comforter for school—I really don't like the pattern or the colors, but I won't let her know. Actually, it's not that important—I shut my eyes when I sleep anyway."

Earnesto Solorzano provided John moral support, relaying his antics at Rollins College in Florida, where he played on the soccer team that won the State NCAA Division II Championship in 1982.

Zelda Ann Thomas wrote frequently of her activities and progress of her injured arm. She underwent surgery in November. She also wrote that she had been working out with the NCS swimming team at the St. Albans' pool. She spoke of a new boy on the STA team but sadly related that he turned out to be "...too young, still very nice, but too young."

Justin Walker in cold, snowy Vermont continued to forward news of classmates and friends in the New England area. He also reminded John to live life to the fullest and asked if he felt memories of their times together were fading. "Jeez, I hope this doesn't mean we're growing up. That's one thing I never want to do."

Some of the more unique letters came from John's great-grandmother, Marion Burgess, of Union, Maine. They were filled with details of family visits to Maine and visits with her daughter, Sadie Lane. Also included were complete listings of what she had planted in her garden and its progress. She had five kinds of beans, squash, cucumbers, beets, carrots, parsnips, Swiss chard, potatoes, tomatoes, and lettuce. "There are ten bugs for every seed," she wrote. She longed for the family to return to the States and was counting the days. She frequently mentioned the baseball strike since she was an avid Red Sox fan, and wrote, "I'm lucky to be as well as I am!"

John's grandmother also wrote from Maine. She mentioned the allergy season and the television event of the summer—the wedding of Prince Charles and Princess Diana. Visits from her two sons and their families were highlights of her life. A trip to Littleton, New Hampshire, where her friends in Eastern Star honored her, was nostalgic. She had lived and raised all three of her children in the White Mountains of New Hampshire. It would always be home.

*　　　*　　　*

> *Keep fighting the things you have to fight and keep looking ahead not back. I think of you and admire you a lot and wish that I had some of the power you have.*
>
> —*Nichola Barcilon*

*　　　*　　　*

In London, Lieutenant Anthony Daly led a colorful 16-man Blues and Royals detachment of troopers of the Queen's Household Cavalry from their barracks for the daily changing of the guard ceremony at Whitehall. They were a picturesque sight in their blue tunics and white buckskin breeches, with the sun glistening off their plumed helmets and shiny breastplates and their unsheathed swords resting on their right shoulders. The troop with their solid black mounts trotted along Hyde Park's South Carriage Drive while tourists watched. As the regiment's scarlet-and-gold standard came alongside a blue Morris Marina sedan, a bomb placed in the trunk of the car, and probably triggered by remote control, rocked the area with a deafening explosion. The blast sent four—and six-inch nails ripping through the troopers as well as bystanders. Three troopers were killed and 22 troopers and civilians were injured. One of the injured troopers died the following day. In addition, seven of the prized horses were either killed or had to be destroyed. One of the fatalities was their leader, Lieutenant Daly. He had been married less than a month and had just returned from his honeymoon in Bermuda with his lovely bride. In one horrible instant, his bride of three weeks had become a widow—nee Nichola Barcilon.

A little over two hours later in nearby Regent's Park, a second bomb exploded under a bandstand where a military band of the Royal Green Jackets was giving a lunchtime concert. Six soldiers were killed and 28 persons were injured.

Bob Barcilon wrote:

Group Captain R.L. Barcilon, AFC RAF
Aylesbury
United Kingdom

August 13, 1982

My Dear John,

I've been meaning to write to you for some time, but I never thought that when I got down to it, it would be in such circumstances. Thank you for your letter—we were all, and Nichola especially, very touched by what you said. Also I suppose (if I can take a quick swipe at you!) we appreciate it particularly as I suppose you don't write too many letters too often!

Seriously, I don't need to tell you what it has been like these past days. I don't know how much you heard or saw in Sweden, but Nichola's personal tragedy was made all the worse by the very public circumstances of Anthony's death, and the fact that his death was pure murder, nothing less. As you know, Nichola is just 24 and had been married less than a month. Anthony was leading his troop of cavalry on ceremonial duty through London when the IRA triggered a 20-pound car bomb alongside him. Thank God, he never knew what hit him—he was dead before he left the saddle.

The whole world knew about it within hours—although I myself was some hundred miles out over the sea in my Lightning when I was recalled to base with no explanation. I then had a four-hour drive home, having picked up the details on the phone after landing.

Well, of course everything went public very quickly, and before we knew it we were all over the papers and the TV. One result was hundreds and hundreds of letters, many from complete strangers, who were so appalled by it all that they had to sit down and write. We are answering them all.

It's very difficult to answer the question, "But why, Daddy?" which poor Nichola kept asking in the days which followed. Neither she, nor poor Anthony, deserved such a thing, and it is very hard to see any purpose in such murderous cruelty. Well, it's been three weeks now, and we are holding together, I suppose, as you would expect, knowing us. Nichola is back home with us, and right now is sitting quietly listening to John Denver and putting photos of her honeymoon into her album. She is mending slowly a little more each day, and now and then we see that lovely smile flash across her face, as we used to so often. The crying has almost stopped now, and with the promise of her own puppy to bring up (Jacquie is thinking about sending all her favorite furniture and fixtures to store while the thing grows up!) she is looking forward again, instead of back.

It's had an effect on all of us, just as your own accident had a major and irreversible effect on your own folks, and we are only now starting to realize how tired and drained we are. Next week I am taking the whole gang down to the coast, for a complete break, and Jacquie needs it as much as anyone.

I suppose this has made us an even closer family than before, if possible. We went to see the wounded troopers in the hospital, and Nichola also saw the wounded horses and even another young girl who also lost a very new husband in the same attack. Two days after Anthony's death, she stood at the same spot where the bomb went off and cheered on the troopers as they went about their normal ceremonial duties—she was caught by the TV and that was even more publicity. And she said to me, "I just won't believe he's not going to walk through that door unless you take me to see him," so I did. I don't need to paint that picture for you I'm sure.

Well, it's all made us a bit selfish, and I apologize for not asking straight away how you are and how things are going for you. I was in the Royal Air Force Club a month ago (for Nichola's wedding) and bumped into Douglas

Bader. We had a longish chat, mostly about you and he was pleased to hear you were ruining legs by tearing around squash courts and generally behaving irresponsibly. He was delighted, in fact. When I told him your age, he just grinned and said, "I was the same age when I made a complete fool of myself. You learn to live with it." Anyway he sends his best wishes. Nice man.

Please give Joanne and your folks our fondest love, and thank them for thinking about us. One day, someplace, we'll meet up again, and it will be like yesterday. That's the true mark of friendship.

True, my friend?

As ever,
Robert

* * *

After a couple of weeks of farewell parties, the Turnover Reception was held at the Embassy on September 20, 1982. Colonel and Mrs. John Forrester were officially introduced to the attaché community and the Swedish military, although Colonel Keating and Colonel Forrester had made formal calls on the military attachés and the Swedish military the preceding week. It was a happy but poignant time for the Keatings. They were going home, but were leaving behind some very dear friends who had shared, on a daily basis, the trials and triumphs of the past 18 months. Dr. and Mrs. Waldemar Skogs and Dr. and Mrs. Lars Hakelius traveled down from Uppsala to attend the reception and wish "the American" and his family the very best in the future. Isabelle, whom John had dated since Midsummer '81 and who had been a frequent houseguest of the Keatings, attended and represented the many wonderful nurses who had been so instrumental in his recovery. Dr. Basil Finer was unable to attend but had been a dinner guest of the Keatings several weeks previous.

* * *

Friday morning arrived and as the Keatings prepared for their flight home, they could not help but reminisce about the times they had shared in Sweden. It was a wonderful assignment, and the friends they had made would become lifelong friends. It is always sad to leave friends but, then again, they were going home! The last 18 months had been most difficult. It was a period which they not only endured but one in which they triumphed. There was a sense of finality, the end of a chapter in their lives. Returning home together had become a goal, and now that goal was about to be attained.

The doorbell interrupted their thoughts. Tord had arrived to drive them to Arlanda where the DAO office personnel, along with Isabelle and the Hammarskjolds, were gathering to bid the Keatings farewell and God speed. It would be a most difficult time for Mike and Judy because Mike's office had been so supportive during this most trying time. Mike and Judy hated to say goodbye to these fine people, but the time had come.

Tord seemed to epitomize the DAO. After all, he had enjoyed a professional relationship with the attaché office for over 30 years as well as being emotionally involved in John's tragedy. He had shared the pain and anguish the Keating family had endured as well as their triumphs because that was the type of caring individual he was. Saying goodbye to Tord would be most difficult.

"Are these all the bags?" Tord asked nodding towards the bags in the hall.

"That's all of them," Mike responded.

Tord began loading the Mercedes. When he had finished, he returned announcing, "They're all loaded. We're ready to go any time."

Judy descended the stairs and greeted Tord. At the foot of the stairs, she glanced one last time back at the house.

Reading her face Tord asked, "You're glad to be going home?"

Judy sighed as if relieved of some heavy burden. "Oh, yes, Tord," she said quietly, "I am."

*　　　*　　　*

We could feel "America the Beautiful" and "America the courageous" through our association with your family during the last two years.

—Koeng-ho Chong

*　　　*　　　*

Epilogue

The Keating family returned to the United States in late September 1982. After reuniting with Grandma Lane and Great Grandma Burgess in Maine and Judy's brothers and their families in Massachusetts and New York, they journeyed to Washington, D.C., where they visited the Hawleys, Singers, Cronins, and McHargues. They visited St. Albans School and talked with Cannon Martin, the Mullins, and members of the faculty. They also were able to visit the Pecks in Texas and the Dunns and Goldens in Georgia before Mike reported for duty at Maxwell AFB, Alabama. Thanksgiving of 1982 was spent in Wisconsin with the Keating side of the family. The reunions were emotionally uplifting and essentially brought closure to the ordeal that had consumed them for the past 18 months.

John enrolled at Auburn University at Montgomery (AUM) and graduated three years later with a degree in Business Administration. Joanne completed high school and began working as a volunteer at a daycare/preschool center. Judy began a counseling career specializing in victims of abuse. Mike retired from the Air Force in 1986 and the family settled in Montgomery, Alabama.

In 1986, John met Melynda Howell of Greenville, Alabama, Mary Cronin's hometown. Melynda was also an AUM graduate. They were married in July of 1988 and settled in Mobile, Alabama, where Melynda taught school. They subsequently moved to Montgomery where Melynda continued her teaching career. They were blessed with three wonderful boys, John Lane, Michael Asa, and Kris Gabriel.

The Keatings have continued to enjoy warm friendships with many of the individuals and families through the intervening years through phone calls, letters, and visits.

Cousin Mike Keating is married and the father of two girls. He and his wife, Karen, live in San Francisco. Dave Singer is married with one child and is president and CEO of a pharmaceutical company in San Francisco. Billy Mondale is a lawyer working in the Minnesota Attorney General's Office. Tom Liddy is running for Congress in Arizona's 1st District.

Isabelle Pettersson visited the Keatings in the United States twice, once during the summer of '83 and then again in the summer of '87. She is still working as a nurse at the Academic Hospital in Uppsala.

Tim and Caroline Puntan are both married and living in England. Tim is the father of twins and Caroline the mother of five. Nichola Barcilon remarried, is the mother of two, and is busy raising a family in England.

Afterwords

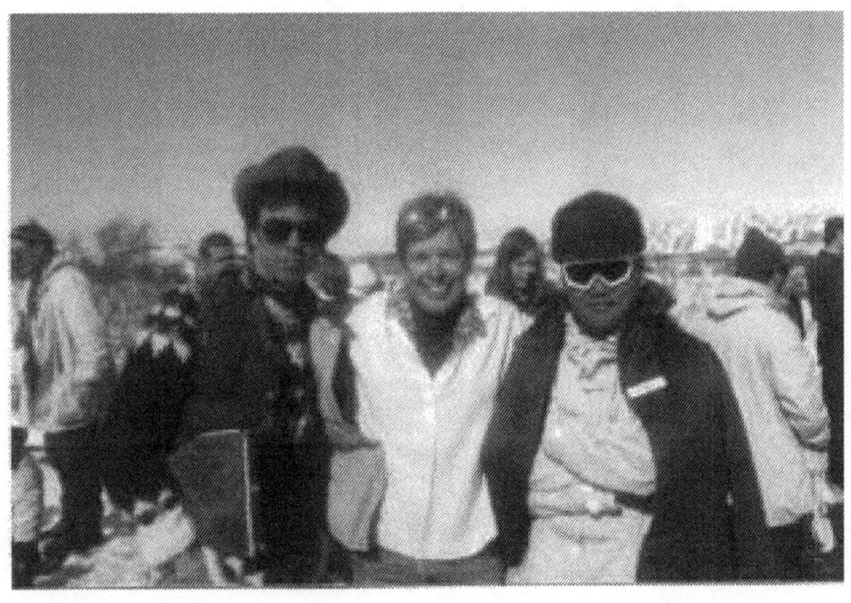

The Attachés complete their trek and are met by the families. John and Judy pose with Tom Yamaski.

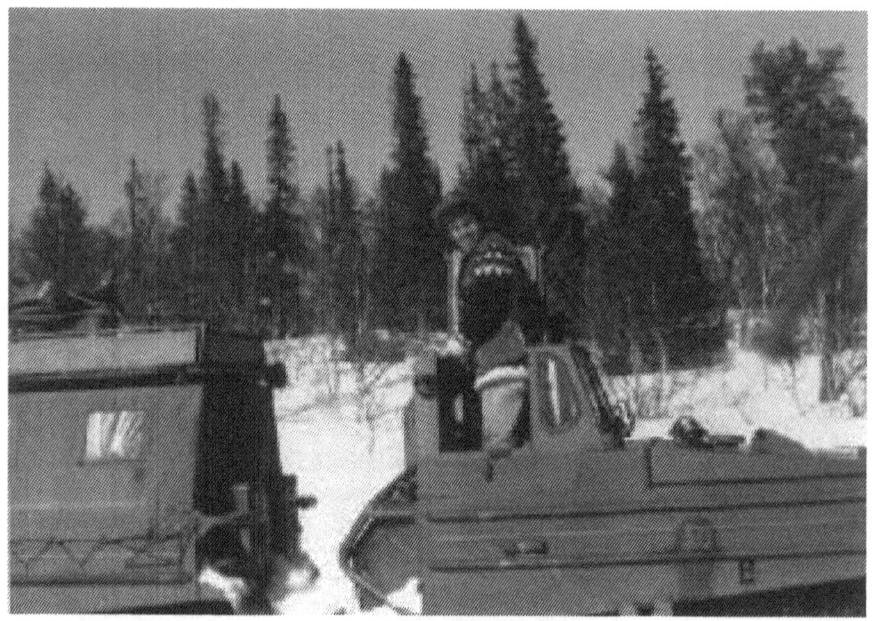

John inspecting a Swedish Army track vehicle.

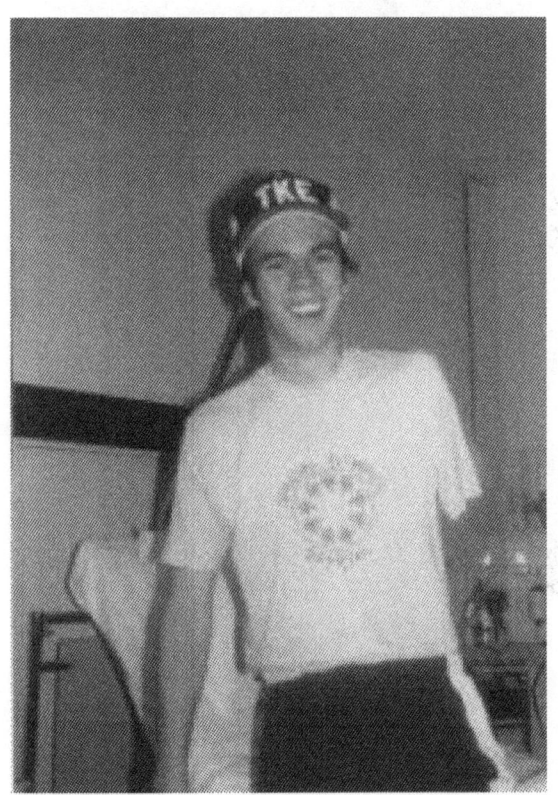

John stands for the first time by himself on May 19, 1981.

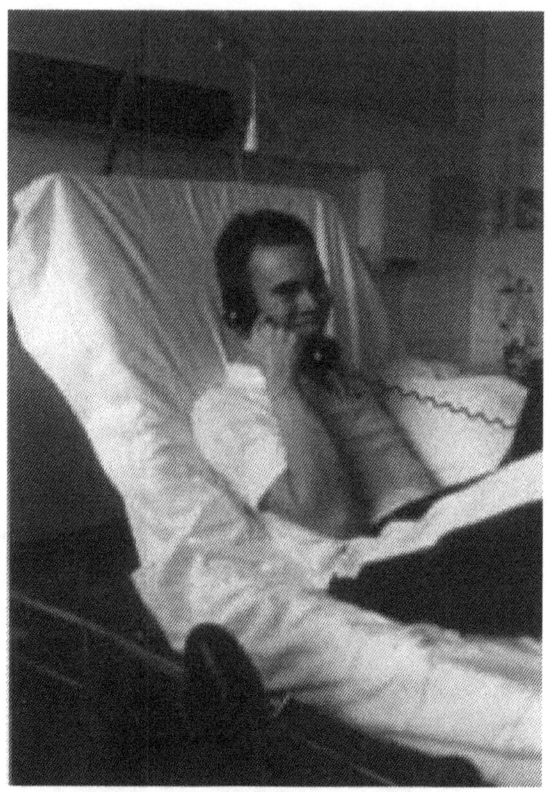

John on the phone with Billy Mondale, Dave Singer, and Carl Cosimano, May 30, 1981.

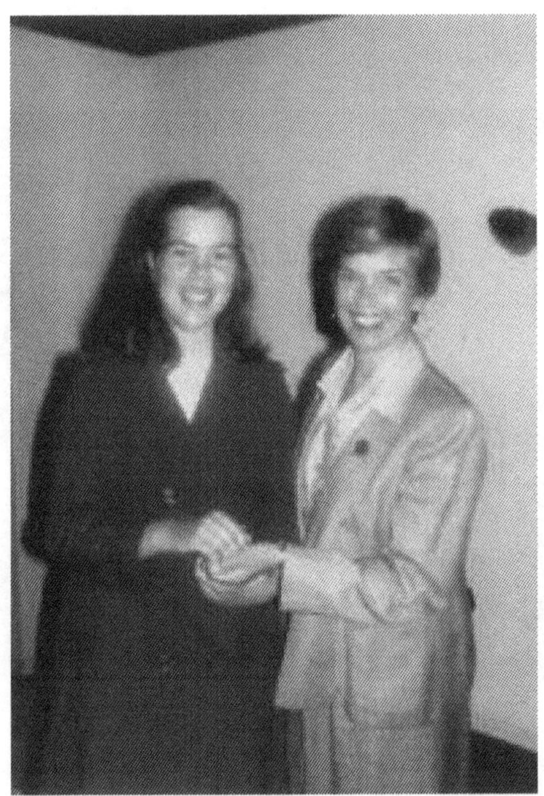

Joanne and her mother admire the ring given to her by her parents for her graduation from the International School.

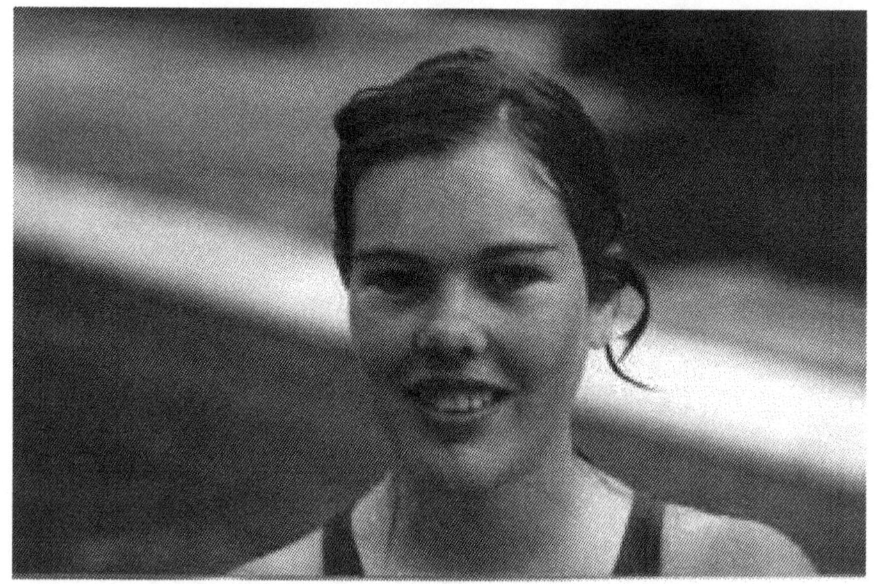

Joanne after a relaxing swim.

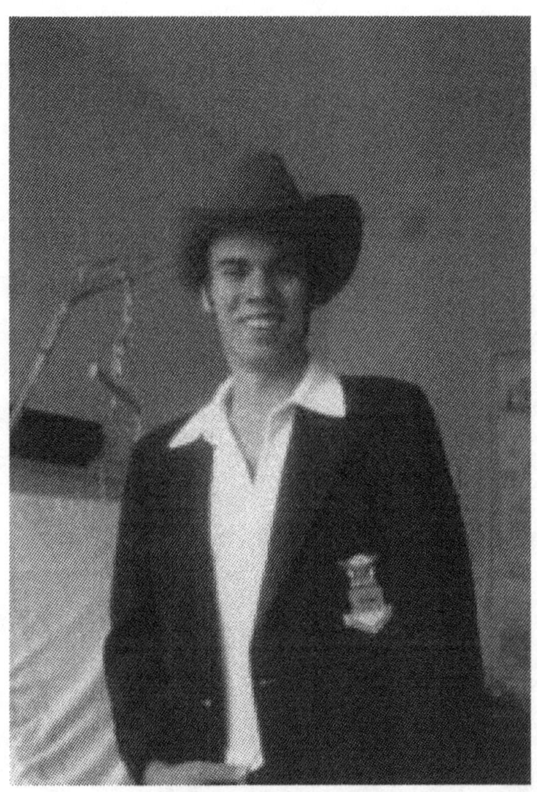

Jonh and his cowboy hat.

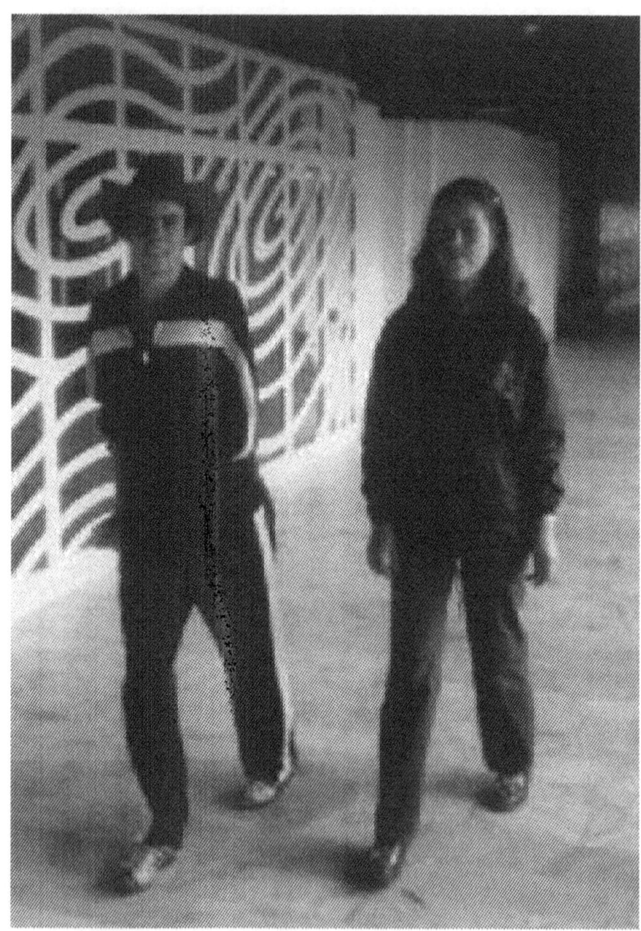

John and Joanne take a short walk, June 6, 1981.

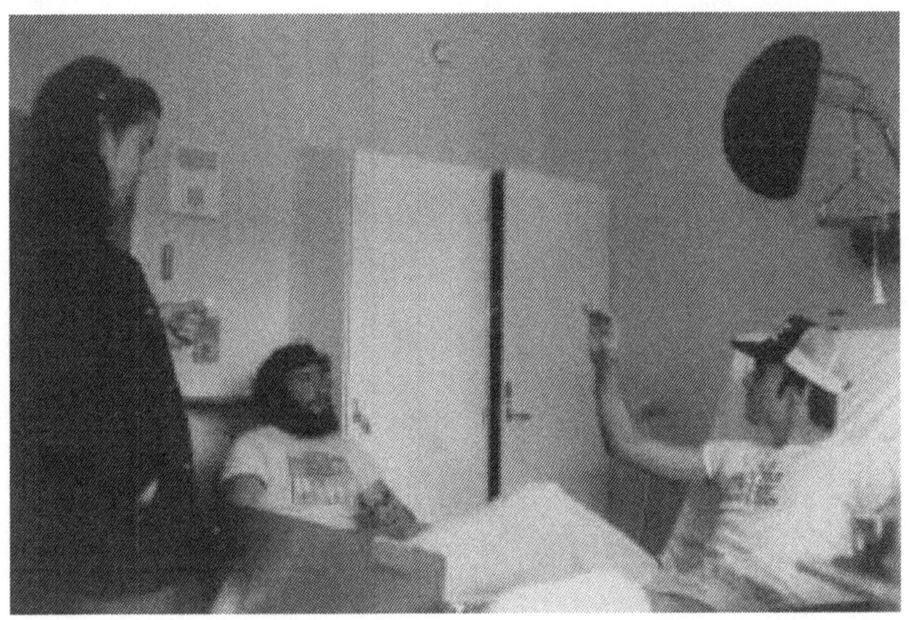

Joanne and cousin Mike visiting John in Uppsala.
Note the cowboy hat hanging from John's pull-up bar.

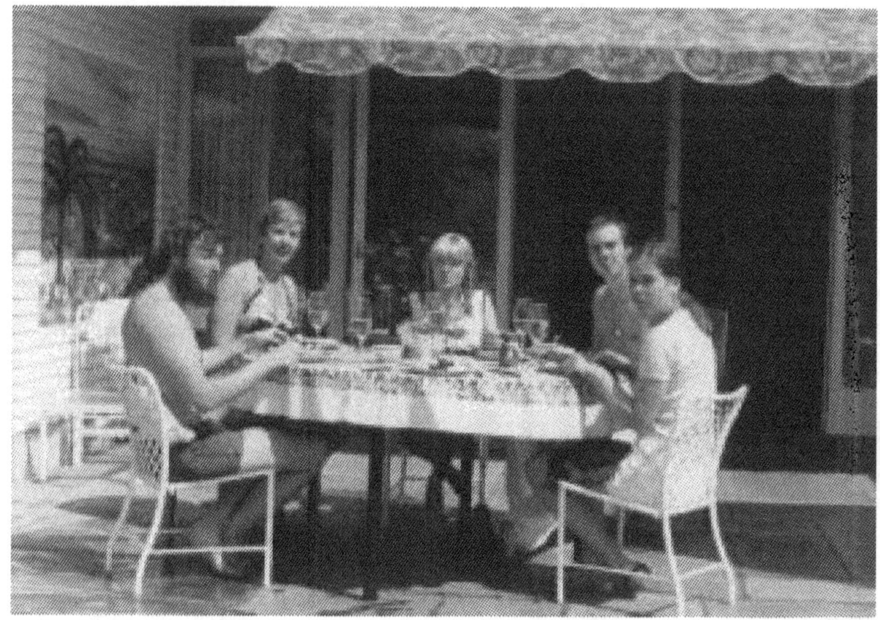

The first day of the Midsummer weekend.
Cousin Mike, Judy, Isabelle, John, and Joanne.

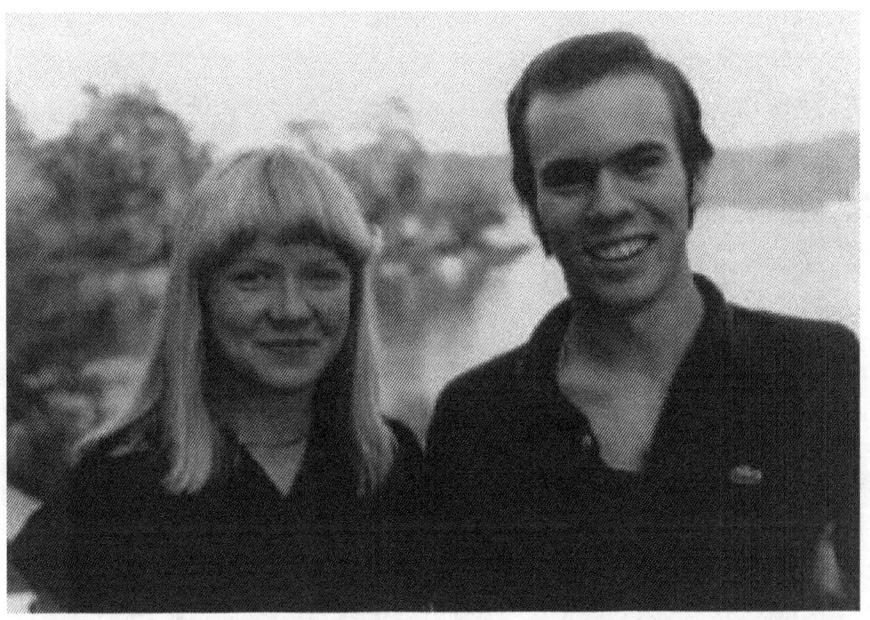

Isabelle and John, Midsummer 1981.

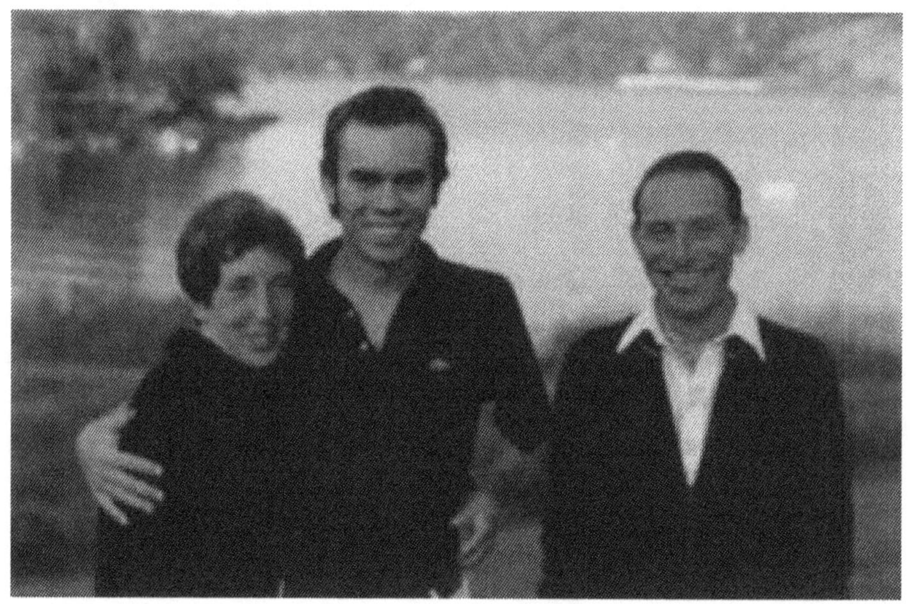

John with Jacquie and Bob Barcilon, Midsummer 1981.

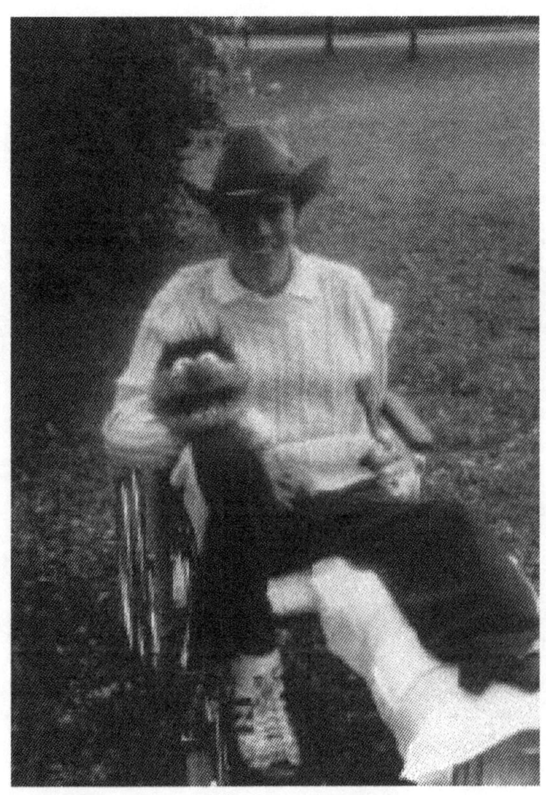

John and Animal picnicking on the hospital grounds.

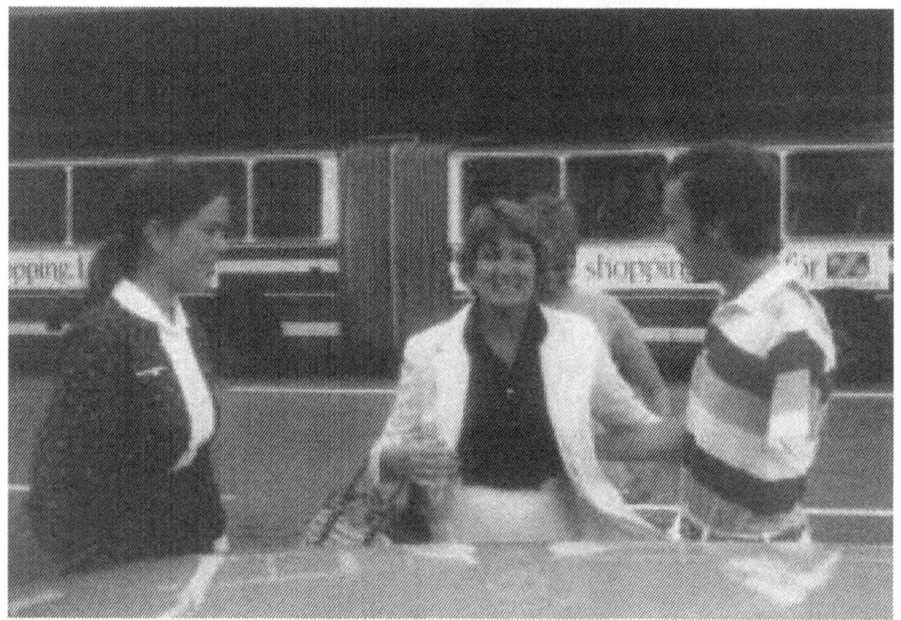

Suzy finally arrives at Arlanda.

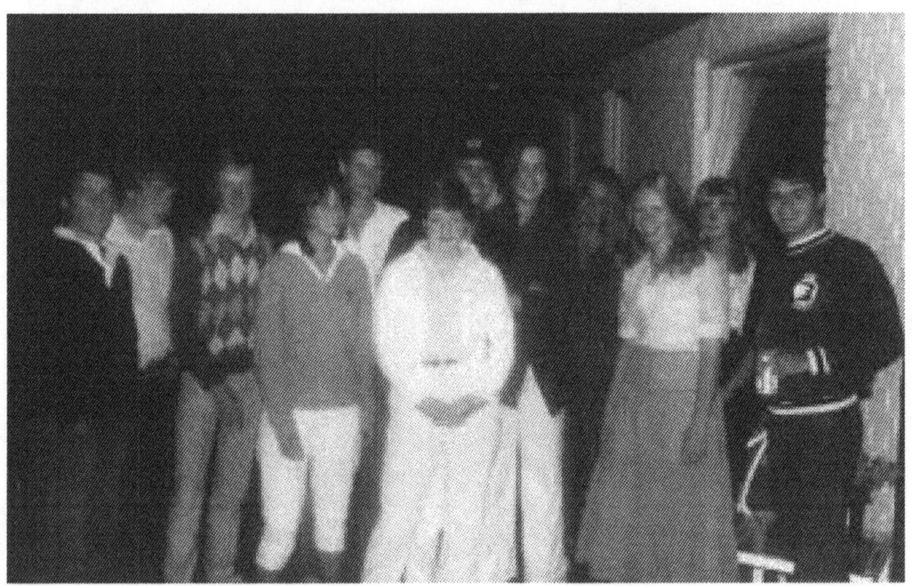

John's Birthday Party. From the left: Dave Singer, David Moss, Tim Puntan, Helena Hokanson, Bobby Thomson, Caroline Puntan, John, Joanne, Beth Thomson, Vivete Olson, Asa Thoden, and Billy Mondale.

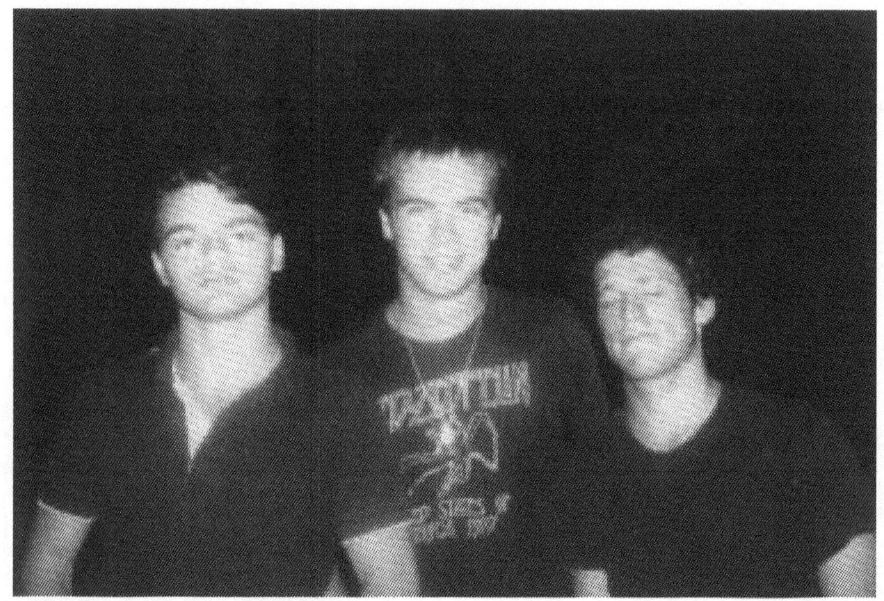

Billy, John, and Dave.

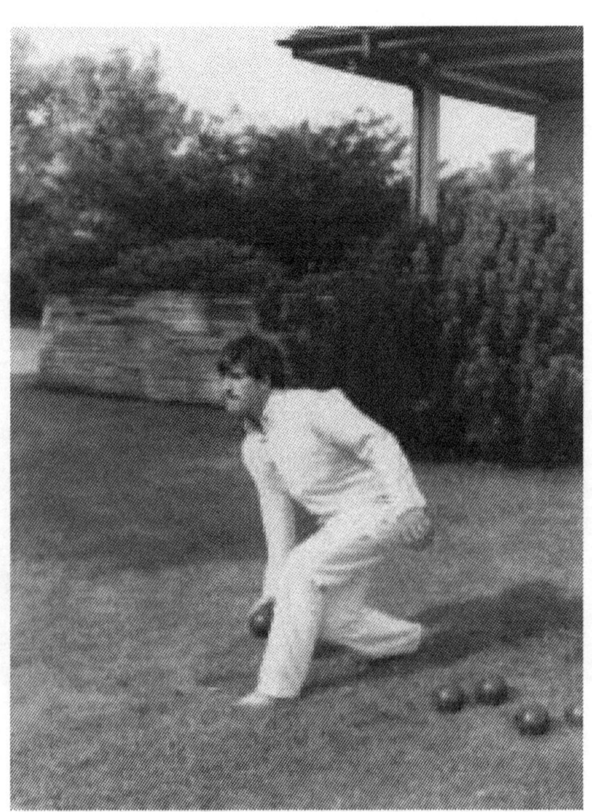

Tom Liddy playing Bocci

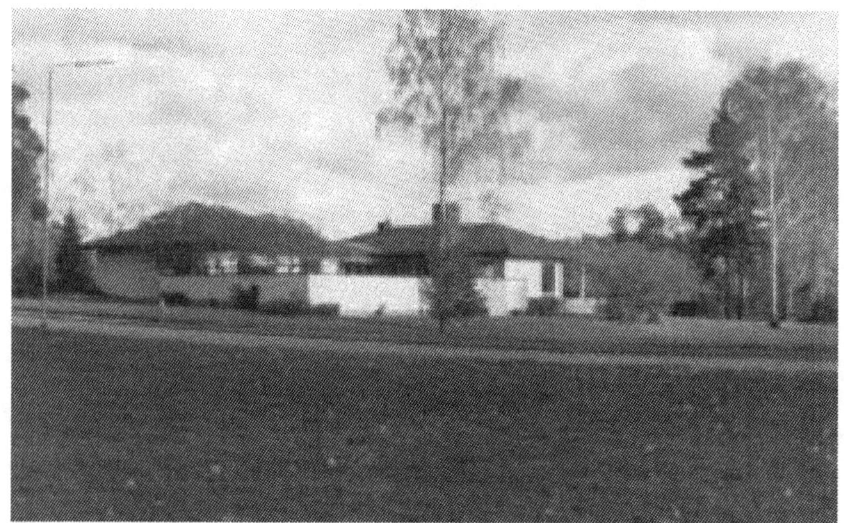

The Keatings' home in Djursholm

Appendix

Letters from 1981

R 092035Z APR 81
FM HQ AFIS FT BELVOIR VA//INK
TO USDAO STOCKHOLM SWEDEN
UNCLAS
FOR COL KEATING FROM COL STEINMILLER
SUBJ: INJURY TO SON OF DATT

WE ARE DEEPLY SADDENED TO LEARN OF JOHN'S ACCIDENT. OUR THOUGHTS AND OUR PRAYERS ARE WITH YOU AND YOURS DURING THE TRYING TIMES AHEAD. PLS ADVISE IF WE CAN BE OF ASSISTANCE.

*　　　　*　　　　*

Embassy of the United States of America
Stockholm, Sweden

April 10, 1981

Dear Judy,

I have just heard the dreadful news about your son. Alan joins me in expressing our sincere sorrow and concern for him and all of you. Please call on us if there is anything we can do and know that our prayers are for your family.

Sincerely,
June Tapsell

* * *

Embassy of the United States of America
Stockholm, Sweden

April 10, 1981

Dear Judy,

Just a note to express our best wishes to all of you and let you know we're thinking of you at this difficult time.

We return from Karlskrona on Wednesday, the 15th, and hope you'll let us know how we might be helpful.

Sincerely,
Beverly Smetheram

* * *

Embassy of the United States of America
Stockholm, Sweden

April 10, 1981

Dear Mike and Judy,

We send our heartfelt sympathy over the truly awful accident that your son had. We pray that with time he will recover fully, and if friendship can be of any assistance, please call on us.

Al & Sue Chapman

* * *

Embassy of the United States of America
Stockholm, Sweden

April 10, 1981

Dear Judy and Mike,

Just to tell you that our thoughts and prayers are with you and John. If there is any way we can be helpful, please let us know.
Our sincere and good wishes,

Ed & Elly Cohen

* * *

Maire and Heikki Tillander
Finnish Embassy
Stockholm, Sweden

April 12, 1981

Dear Judy and Mike,

We want to express our deepest sympathy because of the tragic accident you again had in your family.

Please know that in our hearts and in our prayers we hope that everything would, however, turn out successfully. And that you would have strength to encourage your son.

Sincerely yours,
Maire and Heikki

* * *

Ceci Martin
Alexandria, Virginia

April 12, 1981

Dear John,

We love ya! And you have everyone's support behind you. I wish I could give you more but all I can give ya is my love, my faith, and the best of luck in the world.

Love,
Ceci

* * *

Bitsy Cronin
University of Alabama
Tuscaloosa, Alabama

April 12, 1981

Dear John,

I just wanted to write you to let you know how sorry I was to hear of your accident. Laing called me just tonight to tell me about it, but I had no idea you'd even left school. It seems like ages since I've talked to you. I wish you'd kept in touch; I've missed you so much! Anyway, I really am sorry to hear about this, John. I just wanted you to know that we all love you and we're all behind you always.

School has been treating me well lately, my grades aren't too good (have they ever been?), but I've been working harder than I ever have. I'm doing a lot with my photography class. I absolutely adore it! I'm even thinking of majoring in art with photography emphasis. History is hard, and I'm practically flunking English—it's really giving me a lot of problems towards my grade point average. You won't believe this, but I'm taking French and absolutely loving it! Never thought I'd say that!

Kim Ryne and Lee Wallace say "hi." Hunt is doing great and also says "hi." She had an operation on her knee about two months ago and has been letting me drive her new car. I talked to Jud tonight and he said to tell you he loves and misses you very much. He's gonna be in D.C. all summer again, and I hope by some chance in some way we can all get together again like we used to. I miss that terribly.

Well John (Batman), I just wanted you to know that I'm pulling for ya, and I know everything will work out. Please let me know how you're doing because we're all so concerned. Say hello to your parents and Joanne. Mom, Dad, and Liz send their love. Please take care.

Love,
Bitsy

*   *   *

Embassy of the United States of America
Stockholm, Sweden

April 13, 1981

Dear Judy and Mike,

We have spent a lot of time thinking about you and praying the last few days. I don't know, frankly, how much you would appreciate a call at this time, so I decided to write to you instead. Like any mother of teenagers I am very aware of the fact that what has happened could just as easily have happened to our family and to our child and I hope that we will some day know why it has to happen at all.

I can well understand that Joanne wants to be close to home at this time. We will be back on Easter Monday and any time you want Joanne to spend the night, or weekend, or whatever we would be pleased to have her.

Although I have only personally met John a few times I feel as though I know him quite well. Our son Michael talked a lot about him; Christina volunteered that he was " a neat brother" when she returned from spending the night at your house, and many people around the Embassy have commented on what a nice young man he is.

I guess I just want you to know we are thinking about you and if we can help in any way we are more than willing.

Sincerest regards from our whole family to all of you.

Vanja Huth

* * *

Joanne Golden
Montgomery, Alabama

April 13, 1981

Dear Judy and Mike,

No words can convey our shock concerning John. When Johnny answered your phone call, Mike, the color went out of his face and he sat down in the chair. I knew something dreadful was wrong but never this. Our thoughts and prayers are with you constantly. I wish we were closer. I don't know what we could do but at least be near you.

Johnny taped two tapes of country and western music from WLWI complete with the commercials, news, etc. We thought it would give John something to listen to in the hospital. If it works out and he enjoys them, let us know. We can always do more. He might like rock more than country & western. Just let us know. Johnny went to see General Umstead, told him and gave him your addresses that I had written down. He was as shocked as we were.

Johnny also saw Colonel Hackworth and Mike; he asked to give you a message. He is going to become the Dean of AWC effective in June. He said if you would like to, he would be pleased for you to return to AWC after your Stockholm tour to teach or maybe be head of a department.

Elizabeth is fine. She's grown like a weed this year. Johnny is spending as much time, as the books (and me??) will allow, fishing on Lake Jordan. A week and a half ago he caught 40 fish there in about five hours of fishing. Thank Heaven the limit is 10. I don't see how we could eat 40 fish by the time we leave.

Please keep us informed about John. Give Joanne a hug and a kiss.

Love,
Joanne

* * *

James P. Keating, Jr.
Neenah, Wisconsin

April 13, 1981

Dear Judy & Mike,

Thanks for the call last Saturday, hopefully and collectively we can help John recover from his accident.

It'll take awhile for him to accept that it ***really*** *happened and that he is not just dreaming. That will be a key pivotal point—when he accepts it then makes the decision to forge ahead. It's a miracle he survived; therefore, God must have important plans for John's future. Knowing this, we need to stress future plans, goals, dreams, and aspirations with John.*

Please drop us a note on his progress and we'll do what we can from this end to help John.

Love,
Pete & Sally

* * *

Karen Williams Thomsen
Niagara, Wisconsin

April 13, 1981

Dear Mike and Judy,

We have just heard of John's tragic accident. We know that there is little that we can say or do for you at a time like this, but out thoughts, love and prayers are with you for his recovery.

Love,
Karen

* * *

Mrs. John T. Lane
West Rockport, Maine

April 13, 1981

Dear Judy, Mike, Joanne & John,

We all love you and are thinking of you and wish we could help in some way. We are so far away and no way to talk.

Jack called Sunday night after a weekend at work. Alfred called last night. We are all so upset, but what can we do?

I feel for you, Judy and Mike! How is John taking it? I'm so glad Al brought him here before going to Sweden. We enjoyed his visit so much. I'm glad I sent cookies to him at UNH. I still have more recipes to make so guess you will have to do the cooking.

Get a pet of some kind for him. I wonder about magazines. What would he like? Whittets have been nice to me and suggested mentioning the Kennedy boy who lost his leg and how well he is doing.

Al said send cards but how about jigsaw puzzles or others. It's cold here—30 degrees. My cat is comforting—so cuddly. John had fun with her.

How is Joanne? She can be a big girl now and help John.

Do write and tell us about what happened. My heart is breaking for you.

Love,
Mom

* * *

Sandra Lane
Rosendale, New York

April 13, 1981

Dear Judy and Mike,

We were totally stunned after Mike's call Saturday evening. We all feel so terrible for John. There just aren't words to express what we are feeling for all of you.

I know you'll have to turn all your strength and energy in a positive direction to help John through the next weeks and months ahead. It seems that you and Mike have had too many times when you've been pushed to the limits emotionally. You both seem to possess an unbeatable spirit and courage, but I wish we weren't so far away so we could lend some support at a time like this. Jack made some comment about getting a military flight to go to Sweden. I think the distance makes him feel so helpless, and we would all like to do something to help.

Jack just started his new job with the Army—it will be a three-year tour. He likes it so far—but he's only been on the job for three or four weeks.

I know you will be very busy, but whenever you have a chance please let us know how John is doing and also what his address is.

Please know that our hearts are filled with compassion and love for you all and our thoughts and prayers are with you continually.

Love,
Sandra, Jack & boys

* * *

Beaz and Carrington Wise
Bethesda, Maryland

April 13, 1981

Dear Mike and Judy,

Carrington and I want to express both our sorrow and our support for John and Joanne and for both of you at this time.

We got in touch with the St. Albans School community on Saturday. Their thoughts and prayers are with you all.

Our parish, St. Alban's Parish, prayed for John on Sunday. Suzy tells me that John is in Uppsala in perhaps the world's best burn center.

We pray that something good will come out of Uppsala for John and for you all after this terrible trauma and tragedy. I wish there were something we could do for you directly, but we are keeping you in our thoughts and prayers.

Love,
Carrington & Beaz

* * *

Beaz Wise
Bethesda, Maryland

April 13, 1981

Dear John,

Carrington and I want you to know that we are thinking about you at this very difficult time in your life.

We aren't the only ones. We saw Oscar Brock in church Sunday morning, and he wanted us to convey his warmest greeting and his deepest concerns about your situation. Bob Cain, the St. Alban's chaplain, led our whole congregation in a prayer for you.

About all I know about Uppsala is that good things have come from there. Two great men—Dag Hammarskjold and the head of the Swedish Lutheran Church, who led the world ecumenical movement. Both these men were great because they had the kind of spirit that carried them over overwhelming obstacles. That's precisely the kind of spirit that you'll exhibit in getting through this.

Carrington and I are with you in our thoughts and prayers, along with St. Alban's School and St. Alban's Parish.

Love,
Carrington & Beaz

* * *

Jacquie Barcilon
Lidingo, Sweden

April 14, 1981

Dear Judy,

I just feel if I keep writing to you we can be in close contact together. Remember, as each day goes by is a day nearer our goal of getting John well again and on the road to a full life once more.

You are very much in our thoughts and at this state I can do nothing more other than to reassure you of our friendship—true friendship because no matter where we are we will always value you and Mike as our friends. Thanks for my Birthday Greetings.

God bless and take care,

Robert and Jacquie

*   *   *

Poongja and Koeng-ho Chong
Embassy of South Korea
Stockholm, Sweden

April 14, 1981

Dear Judy and Mike,

We are extremely shocked to hear the misfortune that has come to John. It makes our hearts hurt to realize that he is still in serious condition.

We wish him and you, strong courage and enough capability to overcome the difficulty.

Sincerely,
Poongja and Koeng-ho Chong

* * *

John F. McCune
St. Albans School
Washington, DC

April 14, 1981

Dear John,

Gentleman, may your recovery be swift and may your life soon again be filled with "unadulterated good stuff." You certainly deserve no less. I think of you and pray for you often, John.

My very best,
John McCune

* * *

Embassy of the United States of America
Stockholm, Sweden

April 15, 1981

Dear Mr. & Mrs. Keating,

We would like to express our deep sympathy and concern for you over the most unfortunate accident. We pray for you to the Love of God to help alleviate your pains.

May God, Guardian Spirits and Deities be with you always.

The Kuniyuki family

* * *

The Chaplain
Anglican Church of St. Peter and St. Sigfrid
Stockholm, Sweden

April 15, 1981

Dear Col. and Mrs. Keating,

We have met on a few occasions and so when your many friends at our church told me of recent events in your family I was able to have your family in my mind's eye.

We mentioned you all in our family communion, (discreetly, and without any details that would cause you embarrassment) in our intercessions.

I remembered you as I celebrated the Communion and those of us who know you here are certain that you will be surrounded and strengthened by God's love for you all.

I gave thanks too! As a doctor I know that a miracle saved your son's life. If you really feel low or bad, fasten on the love and concern of your friends and know that you will be in our thoughts and prayers in the challenging days ahead.

The message of Easter is that hope is born out of despair and the darkness.

My love and prayers and God's blessing to you all,

Christopher Frey

* * *

Daniel M. Singer
Washington, D.C.

April 15, 1981

Dear Keatings –

I wish somehow we could reach out to touch you—somehow to hold your hands as a comfort to you and to us.

Through one of Maxine's colleagues at NIH—who has friends at Uppsala Hospital—we got a very upbeat report indicating John is out of danger and that his kidney and cardiac functions seem okay. That's encouraging and hopeful. Also, the report was that the doctor in charge of John's case is one of the world's best and that the burn unit is outstanding. We've been in touch with Suzy Hawley regularly to exchange info. and that's a good clear channel in both directions.

We've told John's peers that the best thing now for them is to write letters to John. And I know John has been part of the prayers at both STA and NCS. If we can do something more, please, please just ask.

Dan

* * *

Ellen Singer
Swarthmore College
Swarthmore, Pennsylvania

Chin Up!

John,

Just a little note to let you know I'm thinking about you. Spring has sprung here, but so has all the work. I have one week of classes and two of exams left. Then back to D.C. for the summer.

Love,
Ellen

* * *

Spud Parker
Landon School
Bethesda, Maryland

April 17, 1981

Dear Mike,

When I heard of John's accident, I knew I wanted to write you, but I am having great difficulty knowing what I want to say. Though we were not close friends, I always think of you with respect for the way you led your life when I knew you and for your unfailing pleasantness. It was a real pleasure for me to see you again while John was at St. Albans and to be reminded of you through him.

Now you and he have suffered a rough blow. I somehow feel that you are better equipped than most to make the best of a bad situation, but that is small consolation. Once again, the uncertainties of life baffle me, and I realize that we must keep pushing on and learning as we go.

My thoughts are with you, Mike, and I desperately hope all goes well.

Best regards
Spud

* * *

Annegret and Bernd von Wagenheim
Embassy of the Federal Republic of Germany
Stockholm, Sweden

April 17, 1981

Dear Judy and Mike,

We are all very concerned about the accident, which happened to your John. We take part with all our thoughts, feelings and good wishes, and we do hope that John is in good hands in Uppsala, where they do everything to relieve his pain and to encourage him.

When we can do something to help you, please phone—we are there.

Yours sincerely,
Annegret and Bernd & Annett and Christian

* * *

Shalini Amerasinghe
National Cathedral School for Girls
Washington, D.C.

April 18, 1981

Dear John,

*I do not expect you to remember me—my name is Shalini Amerasinghe—sound familiar? I am an NCS'er—in the 11th grade. I heard about your accident—so many here were affected by it that those who don't know you (like myself) were affected. Not knowing you—It is hard for me to write—Let's see—Shall I be amusing—No I don't think so—I remember you at your graduation, limping along on crutches...**in your shorts.** Daring boy! I must admit **that** was funny. You're a wild boy aren't you? Do you have a lot of fun?*

*This year's senior class is one big party. They get together on weekdays, weekends and any other time during which they aren't occupied. The BK parties are back in session etc., etc. This is also the time during which college results come back. Horrors. Seriously, it is an awful business. What do you say to one who has been rejected from a college they have wanted to go to since the age of 14? "Oh, too bad. Better luck next time!" No, can't say that can you? It **is** a bummer—of course people create their own misery.*

*If things all seem to be going down hill, they don't have to take you down with them **unless** you allow them too. Everything depends on a person's state of mind. I have had some very rough times—Oh, God. I'm going through some now—but they **won't** get me down because I won't let them. Life is too important to be hindered by the trials. I try to learn through the pain, joy, disgust, and encouragement. Do you agree with this philosophy?*

I am a close friend of Mrs. Pliura—last year's nurse—do you remember her? I gave her the news and she was going to write. You must have received a letter from her by now. I visited her down at Lynchburg. She is teaching (and nursing) at Virginia Episcopal School for Boys. The people there are quite nice.

John, I hope that your spirits are up! Be happy—so easy to say but harder to do! I know, believe me I know—but you can do it. Try. ***Don't give up,*** *whatever you do. I would like to hear from you.* **Do write** *if you find time—just a quick note to tell me how things are going. I will be waiting for your reply.*

Shalini

* * *

Mary Cronin
Bethesda, Maryland

April 18, 1981

Dear John,

This picture is the closest I could find of "Fat Liz"—your best pal! Actually by being fat she can compete with the other "Fat Liz" about town—a-la-Taylor, that is.

Do you think this hat will do justice to the good-looking head of yours? I doubt it but it seemed to beg to be the one chosen. It needed a friend so I hope you will find it compatible. Bitsy tried to describe your hat to me and even sent a picture but apparently—like clothes—hats change in style a bit too. David Singer came by this morning to offer final approval and felt this was a close choice. What do you think? Kit Count (at Count's Western) said he would do whatever John wants.

Listen, I wouldn't think of cooking another Thanksgiving Dinner without you being here—so, if the Cronins are to have turkey—we have to have John. I'm giving you plenty of notice.

By the way "Fat Liz" is on a diet—one meal a day! Can you believe it? No more peanut butter and jelly sandwiches, M&Ms or Fig Newtons—just Cycle 4 and what I slip to her under the table. I'm over being allergic to my shiners and am pleased with my progress. They were tightened yesterday so I'm hitting the aspirin bottle—plus a wine or two. I shock my contemporaries when I smile but so what! I can now boast of a silver spoon in my mouth. And not only that, it's better than the ***Scarsdale Diet!***

Listen again, John—you know you are special to all the Cronins. That's the way it is and always will be. And I want to hear that we are special to you! My Mother called tonight and said to convey her love to John. She always asks about you. Now, John, keep that bright smile on your face—'cause when you're smiling, the whole world smiles with you!

We love you much—Bitsy wants to talk to you and hopes to do that in the coming week.

Lots of cheer from all the Cronins,

Mary, Don, Bitsy, Liz

*　　　*　　　*

John T. Lane
Rosendale, New York

April 19, 1981

Dear Judy, Mike, John, & Joanne,

John—in spite of all that has happened, we can't help but feel that you will get through it all with success greater than any of us can know. We think of you often and wish that you receive our sincere feelings of hope and courage. That goes for all of you guys.

Schedules seem to be constantly changing here. My new job as XO of a General Hospital is proving to be a great challenge and I look forward to the pursuit. However, thirteen to seventeen hour days are a drain to which I am **slowly** *adjusting. Getting time off is difficult, and summer vacations are questionable; so many adjustments in life style are emerging. Alan has been hired as a lifeguard at our local pool—so, he will likely not make it to Maine this summer. Brian is seeking part time work with a "Rent-a-Kid" program, and Sandra continues her part time work in a bank; so, our household is in a state of flux.*

I called Mom this morning and found Grandma Burgess and Alfred and family visiting. We shared, with Mom and Carolyn, news of John's progress. Some correspondence has passed between Alfred and me relative to wills, deeds, etc. Mom has openly expressed her desires—I was surprised and impressed. However, Alfred does not approve because of inequity. The situation is far from resolved. I have taken Judy's advice—these matters are becoming increasingly less important.

Thinking of you—

Love,
Jack

* * *

Alan Lane
Rosendale, New York

April 19, 1981

Dear John,

I am very sorry about your accident and hope you have a quick recovery.

Our football season didn't go so well this year with three wins and six losses. However, wrestling went well for me this year with 12 wins and one loss, in the beginning of the year 13 to 6. All my victories were pins. The loss was against a junior so that next year; I will get another shot at him. It was convenient having my own personal photographer at all my wrestling meets. Her name is Carol and I have been dating her since October.

School is going fair, however, SAT's are coming up in May. Right now I am finishing up a WSI (Water Safety Instruction) course at a nearby college so I will have more qualifications as a lifeguard. I applied at the pool just down the road along with 25 other people a couple months ago, and recently found out I got the job. I am still lifting weights every day. I have sent two tapes of the top 30 songs.

Your cousin,
Alan

*　　　*　　　*

Brian Lane
Rosendale, New York

April 19, 1981

Dear John,

I heard about your accident and really feel bad about it. I hope that you do not have to stay in the hospital too long. Our football team did fairly well this year. I am only in the eighth grade, so we only have five games. Our record was 3-2. My position was right tackle on offense and on defense. I was also on the wrestling team at a weight of 138. My record was 10-0.

There are only about nine weeks of school left until summer vacation. Alan got a job at the pool right below our house as a lifeguard, so he will probably not go with us to Maine. With my father getting a full time job working in the Army up in Albany, we might not spend too much time up there either.

The weather yesterday (4/18/81) was about 80°F, the warmest it has been in a long time. Alan and I put down some Scott's fertilizer on the lawn. There are some yellow stripes going down the lawn where we missed.

I put a couple of coats of paint on the backboard of our basketball hoop so it wouldn't fall apart.

Your cousin,
Brian

* * *

John Davis
St. Albans School
Washington, D.C.

Easter Sunday

April 19, 1981

Dear Mike & Judy,

Please let me know what I can do if—as the summer rolls around—there seems to be a thought that a Washington university like G.W. or American would be possible in light of the therapy facilities here for John.

How wonderful that you have each other in this hard period for everyone!

My affection, and let me know what I can do.

John

*   *   *

Dave Singer
Yale University
New Haven, Connecticut

April 20, 1981

Country,

From what we hear things seem to be looking up for you—lets keep it that way.

School's winding down and the work is piling up. I'll finish everything on the 11th of May. I'm going home, but then I might be going to Texas to pump oil. I'm really excited about going, but part of me would rather be in D.C. with everyone. I don't know what Billy's written you, but no matter where I work, Billy and I are leaving for Europe on July 24th or 25th. We have plans, either to work north from Madrid or work south from Stockholm. In any case, we will be spending some days with you. The way we route the trip really depends on $.

I went home this weekend for Passover. It was exactly what I needed. I spent most of the time with Emily. She is over Kit and we had a really good time. I kinda like the way things are going now, because I don't get depressed when I leave her, but we both have a great time with each other. I dropped by to see Mrs. Cronin and we talked for a while.

We had room draw the other night and Errol drew the King and no one drew the ace so we got the best room. For seven of us, we got five singles, one double and a living room. I'm in the double with Israel. You met those two over Thanksgiving.

Anyway, I gotta get this letter to the Post Office before it closes. Look forward to hearing from you. Chin up.

Love ya,
Starsky

* * *

James P. Keating
Neenah, Wisconsin

April 21, 1981

Dear Judy & Mike:

Just returning yesterday from a short vacation in Sea Island, Georgia, we learned of the tragic accident to dear John. At a time like this, words are scant solace and, although we have no particular details, Katherine joins me in expressing our sorrow at such an unfortunate happening.

I do hope John can be mended to allow a meaningful and productive life and, if anyone can do it, he will.

Please tell John we will hope and we will pray for him to get maximum recovery with the help of God.

Our sincere sympathy.
Jim

* * *

Bosse and Lena Stromgren
Taby, Sweden

April 21, 1981

Dear Judy and Mike,

We just heard from Carol about the terrible accident John had. We were both very shocked when we got the news. All our thoughts and feelings are with you and we fully understand the hard time you are going through right now. Let's all hope for the best for John even though it may look dark now.

If there is anything we can do to help lighten your burden and if we can be your support in some way, please let us know. We'd be more than happy to help.

Love,
Lena and Bosse

* * *

Spike & Marge Briggs
Monument, Colorado

April 22, 1981

Dear Judy and Mike,

Just heard via Patti Curtis about John's horrible accident. You poor dears—what can possibly console you except knowing our prayers are with all of you? Patti didn't know many details, but at this point that's not what's important. I'm sending a page from a very favorite monthly booklet. Mary Mahoney Barrett sent me my first copy of it 13 years ago and I've subscribed every year since. May you be comforted by it too. I pray for John's perfect healing and that his life will be fuller, and more meaningful as a result of this tragedy.

With you in spirit,
Spike & Marge

* * *

Dr. and Mrs. William Feller
Bethesda, Maryland

April 22, 1981

Dear Judy and Mike,

I can't express how sad Bill and I, and all the other FSI teachers, were to hear about John's accident. We were all horrified but at the same time grateful to know that he is recovering. Our thoughts and prayers are with you, and we wish John a speedy recovery, strength and courage.

It is so difficult to accept tragedies like this. Our children are so precious to us and it seems that we spend so much time and energy protecting them, and yet an accident happens so unbelievably fast. We take our safety and well being for granted until an accident occurs and we realize that all that we enjoy is but for the grace of God.

I understand that John is quite an athlete and I'm sure that this will be a very important positive factor in his recovery. We wish him all the best and pray that you may all find hope, encouragement, strength and comfort in our love for one another.

With all our best wishes,
Bill and Margareta

* * *

Sten and Ann Mari Flodin
Stockholm, Sweden

April 22, 1981

Dearest friends,

Sten and I have just learned about your son's terrible accident in Storlien. I phoned the Embassy so we know that the operation takes place today. One can only pray to God that He helps your son and gives you all strength.

We think of you!
Ann Mari

* * *

M/Gen Hans Neij
Embassy of Sweden
Washington, D.C.

April 22, 1981

Dear Judy and Mike,

I was in Stockholm April 6-15 to attend the annual Attaché meeting. The last day just before I returned to D.C., I learned about your son's accident. Both Kerstin and I feel very, very unhappy about this tragic accident. Please, be sure that our thoughts are close to you and your family these severe days.

Your friends,
Kerstin and Hans

* * *

Mrs. James E. Briggs, Jr.
Monument, Colorado

April 23, 1981

Dear John,

Our family sends special thoughts and love to you during what must be a very trying time. We hope your recovery will be rapid and with few if any complications.

I don't really know you as a man—seems like yesterday you were romping around over in the Pleasant View house with the Briggs girls, Snowaerts, Sandforts, etc.—And now Liz (25) is married six years with a baby boy—Courtney just graduated from high school—will go to Univ. of No. Colo. (nursing)—Angela (20) who went through her share of problems will be a junior at Colo. State, majoring in English—Mark (19) will be a sophomore at Texas Tech in Lubbock—Eric will be a senior in high school—Crickett a sophomore and Susan 8th grade. Everyone's busy with jobs here this summer. Mark is living with a guy in Golden—they both work at some place outside of Denver. Eric and Courtney work at the local Village Inn Pancake House and Angela has an apartment in Colorado Springs. I really need a scheduling book as I can't keep up with everyone—someone is coming or going constantly!

I'm sending along my very favorite booklet—to help you through your ordeal. Everyone is probably trying to send things of cheer and humor—I will send something to cheer and encourage (hopefully) your spirit—for when you spirit is cheered you will be on top of things. This booklet is not the usual type—but very positive and very soul filling.

Blessings & healing to you,
Marge Briggs

* * *

General Dick Stenberg
Chief of the Air Force
Stockholm, Sweden

April 24, 1981

Dear Judy and Mike,

Recently informed about the accident your son had during his visit in Sweden I am writing to tell you that Maj and I very well understand the despair you and your family must feel just now. We also understand that the only thing that can help for the moment is proper medical treatment for your son. We are quite sure he will get it.

I know that you also will hear from the chief of my staff that we of course are prepared to help you if there is anything we possibly can do.

Yours sincerely,
Dick

* * *

General Evert Boge
Chief of the Air Staff
Stockholm, Sweden

April 24, 1981

Dear Friends,

Anders Westerlund has informed me about the terrible accident that your son has been involved in.

My wife and I feel deeply sorry for you and your family. Please let us know if we can be of any help to you.

Yours sincerely,
Evert Boge

* * *

Vivian and Bill Buchanan
Orrington, Maine

April 24, 1981

Dear Judy and Mike,

We were deeply shocked and saddened to hear of John's tragic accident. Words cannot tell you how sorry we are for all of you and especially John. We pray he will get along well and be spared any more suffering. He must have gone through a dreadfully, painful ordeal. It must have been nothing short of a miracle that he survived.

We hope he will find the strength and courage, and we're sure he will, to cope with the days ahead.

We had a similar tragic accident here about two months ago. Our next-door neighbors' 19 year-old son was working in the woods and a tree fell on him, breaking his back, and paralyzing the lower half of his body. He is still in the hospital of course having therapy, etc. His mother grew up with Connie and was her closest friend. So we have an idea of some of the agony you are going through.

However, it is said that "God never closes a door without opening a window somewhere." We hope this will hold true for John.

Wanted to let you know we were thinking of you all. I must write a note to your Mother and Grandmother. They must be very upset.

Sincerely,

Vivian & Bill

* * *

Caroline Puntan
Cambridge, England

April 25, 1981

Dear Colonel and Mrs. Keating and Joanne,

Thank you for your phone call on Tuesday evening. It was nice to know that the doctors felt the operation was not urgent, although John must have been not very pleased as he seems, understandably, to want to get it over with.

How is he feeling now? Still in fairly good spirits I hope. I expect you have been up to Uppsala to see him. Have you had any further news about him moving to another ward? If you do please let my parents know so that they can tell me (a good excuse for them to write to me) so I can send him some magazine and letters.

Joanne, how did school go? Did you have to spend the first lesson in the library putting away "dumb books"? Was John's hat found? If not, would you like me to see if I can get one in London? If so, what size do you suggest?

Tim and I had a good flight back on Wednesday morning, and Tim was met at Heathrow by his landlady (some people have all the luck) and I got to Cambridge at about 6:30 pm after accidentally catching the slow train to Cambridge.

Thank you so much for taking us up to Uppsala to see John and thank you also for keeping us informed about his condition.

Love,
Caroline

* * *

Col. and Mrs. P. K. Crowley
Arlington, Virginia

April 27, 1981

Dear Mike and Judy,

For ten days now I have tried to think of what to say to you. I haven't yet figured out what I could say or should say etc., but decided to write anyway and let you know I'm thinking of you in your time of trouble. If anyone in this world is strong enough to see this all through, you're it. And I know John is one who can survive this and "carry on" with success. At nineteen he's a good man.

In less than three weeks I will finish my language course. Then after one week of briefings, Faye and I will return to Tampa for a little vacation before departure to Cairo.

The Goldens will arrive in Tampa on the 4th of June and stay with us until they find an apartment suitable.

Please give John my best regards. Tell him I think of him every day. I do!

Sincerely,
PK

* * *

Jonna Jarnfelt
Espoo, Finland

April 27, 1981

Dear John,

I don't know if you exactly remember me, but we met a couple of times last summer. I lived next door to David Singer and I met you before you went to Sweden. I've been writing to Stephanie, Dave's sister, since I left Washington, D.C., and today I got a letter from her which told me what had happened to you. I thought that I could write you, just because I myself ***love*** *to get letters while I'm ill or anytime. I'm sorry if my English isn't perfect, but I try to write as good as I can.*

It's really stupid to think that far away from this cold and silent country, I have friends with whom I spend last summer. Sometimes I think that they don't exist at all. But every time I get a letter from the States it reminds me that there really are some people out there.

My life is school, friends, dance and family. As you might remember, I speak Swedish with my family and in school, but Finnish with my friends here where I live. I live in Tapiola, a suburb outside of Helsinki, 9 km from it.

To be honest, I really don't know what to write to you about, but I just know that I want you to have my warmest love and my best wishes and if you feel like it, you can write me anytime. ***Be well again*** *and take care of yourself. I hope we will see each other again. My address is on the envelope.*

Love,
Jonna

* * *

Brigit and Anders Westerlund
Stockholm, Sweden

April 27, 1981

Dear friends,

We want to express our deepest sympathy to you and your boy. There is nothing I can say to comfort you that would not sound wrong, so I will just say that we think about you all.

Love,
Brigit and Anders

* * *

Church and Wooz Mathews
Hume, Virginia

hang in there and get well soon

We're all thinking of you and hoping for a speedy rehabilitation. We learned of your accident while in Washington for Kirk's knee operation. He's doing well and we're hoping he will be headed for West Point in July. Best to your parents.

Church & Wooz Mathews

* * *

Earnesto Solorzano
St. Albans School
Washington, D.C.

April 30, 1981

Dear John,

Que pasa brother? I hope you're feeling better. To tell you the truth, I've never written a letter in English, but this one will gladly be the first one. The day that I heard about your accident was the same day Stables, Cafritz, Jamie Sullivan and I were visiting the Bishop's garden and were thinking a lot of you. It was a weird experience.

Here at school everything is boring. I can't wait to get the heck out. I'm sure you know what I'm talking about. All the teachers remember you and were very much shocked when they heard about you.

Now I'm playing lacrosse, and since the first game I have worn your number. But, only when we wear white—because I'm sure you stole the blue jersey. Right now I'm in Omni class (first period) listening to Mr. Eagles talk about Hitler. How are your parents? I hope they are fine. Give them my best regards—also say hello to your sister.

I'm sorry I hadn't written you early, but I really didn't know how to act and what to say to you. But I decided that was stupid and started to write to my favorite Latino **BROTHER**. *John, if there is any way that I could be of any help to you, feel free to tell me and I'll do anything I can to do what you need.*

Man I get so mad that bad things have to happen to people that don't deserve it. All I ask you as a brother is not to get down, instead, my friend be thankful that you can still read this dumb letter that I'm writing to you.

Brother take care. Always your brother,

Love,
Earnesto

* * *

Alyson Denny
Washington, D.C.

April 1981

Hi John,

Basically I just wanted to write to tell you that if you believe that a collective body of people and their faith and love can help you, you sure have it. If I were religious, I would pray. As it is, I will just hope with all my heart that you can deal with your difficult situation. I have much confidence in you!
Good luck,

Love,
Alyson

* * *

Dr. Lee King
Stockholm, Sweden

April 1981

Mr. and Mrs. Michael Keating,

Please add my prayers to the many of those that go heavenward for the recovery of your beloved son and keep your belief that miracles happen every day in this uncertain world of ours. Our true heartbreaks are in our suffering over the uncertain events that happen to our children—this is the heritage of a parent.

There is nothing I can say that will lighten your burden. You do have my love and prayers.

Lee King

*   *   *

Al & Carolyn Lane
Boxford, Massachusetts

April 1981

Dear Judy & Mike,

Needless to say we have been thinking of you and John day and night since his accident. Being related and also parents ourselves brings it all close to home even though we are so many miles away. I hope you can feel that we are all 100 percent behind you, the small comfort that it may bring.

Having had the opportunity to spend more time with John recently was particularly rewarding and fun. We are so fond of him and he has a "reserved" spot of love in our hearts. Seeing his potential, we pray that he can believe in his multi-abilities and strengths to help carry him through this difficult period. He will be a much finer, stronger person than all of us put together in the end, I'm sure.

Thank you for keeping us all posted. We have had several phone calls with Jack and Sandra. Your friend from Virginia was particularly kind to call. After her report, we felt a little more positive than before.

I guess we are all together in spirit. After I finished the previous page of this letter, Mom called and said she had talked with you as you had called. She really appreciated your call. You've been great about keeping us posted. We hang on edge from week to week hoping progress is continuing. We don't expect letters from you with all you have to do. Does John have a tape or cassette? Let us know when you call the States again or we'll call.

Tell Joanne we know what a big help she has been and that we send our love to her also.

Love,
Carolyn

* * *

Ceci Martin
Alexandria, Virginia

April 1981

Dear John,

Hey, Babes! I hear you're not doing so well....Well to that I say, I'm sure you'll be better soon. Everyone over here is supporting you, and I'm sending all my love to you to help you pull through with flying colors.

Well enough on that subject. Listen I wish that you had sent word down this way when you left UNH, cause I was ***really*** *looking forward to seeing you this spring. I was pretty disappointed when Fat Rob told me you went home! So listen you owe me one visit. Next time you're anywhere near this area you better let me know because I want to see ya so damn bad!*

Oh, I got a letter the other day from Susy C. She says to give you a big kiss the next time I see ya so here it is!! I'll give it to you in person next time. Susy is doing fine. I've been paddling a lot this year and am now on the circuit and having a blast. Hopefully I'll make the cuts in May and make it onto the 1982 US Whitewater Team but who knows....

As for my love life, it sucks at this point. I broke up with this paddler I was going out with since Aug. And since then I've been pretty bored, but I hope that will change soon. Let's see what else do I have to tell ya? I really can't think of anything but that I love you and want you to take care. I'm dying to hear from you and am dying even more to see ya.

Love you always and take the best of care.

Ceci
Love & Kisses XXX OOO

* * *

Stu Wood
Littleton, Colorado

April 1981

Dearest Judy and Mike,

Our prayers and thoughts have been with John and you all ever since we heard of his terrible accident. Knowing as little as we do of the facts and current situation, we can but continue praying. With that in mind I offer a segment of a Psalm, which I read in church. Somehow it seems appropriate.

The cords of death entangle me; the grip of the grave took hold of me, I came to grief and sorrow.

Then I called upon the Name of the Lord; "O Lord, I pray you, save my life."

Gracious is the Lord and righteous; our God is full of compassion.

The Lord watches over the innocent; I was brought very low, and He helped me.

Turn again to your rest, O my soul, for the Lord has treated you well.

For you have rescued my life from death, my eyes from tears, my feet from stumbling.

I walk in the presence of the Lord ——

I will lift up the cup of Salvation and call upon the Name of the Lord.

With complete dedication I offer to you all whatever service we may be able to accomplish. Let us know how we can ease your (collective) grief and pain. You can be assured we will do everything in our power. Will your tour there continue as scheduled or will it be—or has it been curtailed? Let us know the developments so that we might be able to render assistance.

What are the plans for John's continued schooling? I (we) would be pleased to research opportunities out here in Colorado. As you are well aware, there are some excellent schools in and near Denver, which John might like.

All of our love, prayers and desires to help,
Pat & Stu

* * *

Maxine Singer
Washington, D.C.

May 2, 1981

Dear Judy and Mike,

You can imagine how thrilled we were to get John's letter yesterday! Stephanie called me at the lab just as soon as she arrived home from school and found it. Two days ago Suzy Hawley called to tell us about her letter too. John sounded as though he had himself well organized—and while I know he will have his ups and downs, he seems to have the strength to proceed well. His big concern was the two of you, as I'm sure you know.

The Singer children are preparing themselves for examination—in New Haven, Swarthmore and at home. Shortly we'll have a full house again while they do their laundry, see friends, refurbish wardrobes and finally they'll disperse for summer jobs, school, trips, etc.

Washington is ablaze with azaleas, but to tell the truth, it's been so chilly and rainy that there hasn't been much time to enjoy it. I went out in our garden earlier this morning, but my fingers were frozen in five minutes.

All the best,
Maxine

*   *   *

Chuck & Patti Curtis
Colorado Springs, Colorado

May 5, 1981

Dear Judy and Mike,

Bari & Dan will be here next week—and we shall be talking of you—and remembering you—and wishing we were there to give you some solace—or cheer.

Bari mentioned after her phone call to you that John was off his life support machines. We hope that his progress is miraculous—for all your sakes.

Since we are incapable of helping you—we only want you to know we care—and suffer with you.

If you ever feel like writing, we'd love to hear from you. But we'll keep in touch no matter what via the grapevine of mutual friends. I cannot remember your friend (with twins?) here—the widow. Marge Briggs and I both lost her name somewhere.

We send our wishes of speedy recovery to John and for strength and love to you—
Patti & Chuck

*   *   *

Col. and Mrs. David Penniman
Dover, New Hampshire

May 5, 1981

Dear John,

Our thanks to Danny for stopping by with news from the Keatings; however, we are sorry that it had to be bad news. We are truly sorry, John, to hear of your accident. It seems you have had more than your share of doctors and hospitals in the last few months! You are young and strong so we know you will make a speedy recovery. Keep smiling with that chin up.

We are thinking that spring might actually come to this area after all. Things are getting green and leaves are popping. Sure seems slow compared with Montgomery. The girls write from Alabama that it's 85°F and they're sunbathing!

UNH is into the whirl of end-of-year activities. Students are gearing up for final exams starting the end of next week. The grand finale will be graduation, May 24.

We will be leaving for Montgomery on June 1 barring unforseens to attend Linda's graduation from Troy State. She is job-hunting now with not much success so far. Karen will finish her finals on June 8 at Auburn and return to NH with us for the summer. We expect Linda will remain in Alabama. Another Yankee lost to the South!

We have been keeping very busy working in the yard. Hope soon to have the driveway paved. Dave is also waiting for a load (7 cords) of true length timber for the stove next winter. Life is different!

We hope things are looking up for all of you and that things will be reasonably normal soon.

Sincerely,
Nancy

* * *

Stephanie Singer
Washington, D.C.

May 5, 1981

Dear John,

Thank you for your letter!! It's so exciting to find it in the pile with all the junk mail, bills, and alumni committee sendings—many letters. "Sweden" was a refreshing postmark.

Last Wednesday we took a field trip to Capitol Hill. Sue Simpson's father is a Senator and he got us a tour of the Dome. The stairs were very steep and narrow and some people got sick, but the view at the top was incredible. The whole city is visible and I really got the feeling that all the roads lead to the Capitol. It was a sense of being absolutely, incredibility in the center of the city.

Because of the field trip, I didn't find out until today about the English paper due tomorrow and the typewriter broke. (I've learned to type and I type **everything** *now—except personal letters.) So the paper will have to wait a couple of days.*

We talked to Dave the night before his Biology exam. He sounded happy and not too worried about studying.

Love,*
Steph

**2 cups admiration*
2 cups strength
Stir. Sprinkle with genuine sisterly affection. Serve boiling hot.

* * *

Zelda Ann Thomas
Washington, DC

May 5, 1981

Dear John,

How ya doin? I shouldn't be writing you because you never wrote me. But I've been thinking of you especially now that it's spring and exactly a year ago we were going out.

I hope you're feeling better. I sort of know how you feel, because, I don't know if I ever told you, but I had an accident where I fell through a glass door and severed all my nerves. My arm is partially paralyzed and I'm in the middle of a suit against the glass company for the negligence they portrayed by putting in this cheap glass, which hurt me so bad!

I know you'll come through though! I was glad to hear you were still your old self—checking out the cute Swedish nurses, m m m !

I haven't seen you for so long! I truly think about you a lot, I was so bummed I didn't get to see you when you were here during Thanksgiving! I hope you'll come visit me this summer, or even better, come steal me away from prom night! Please help me!

I haven't written Bitsy for a long time but I presume you've heard from her! I hope you're feeling good enough to write! You'd better!

Please, please write me back and tell me how you're doin! Maybe sometime this summer you can come visit. Mom's a lot more lenient about things this year! She even lets me go out past 10:30—ha, ha! No, she is nicer!

Well, write me please!

All my love,
Zelda

*   *   *

Embassy of the United States of America
Stockholm, Sweden

May 6, 1981

Dear Judy & Mike,

I would like you to know how very much you have been in our minds over the past days. The day I heard of your son's accident I was reminded of the pain I felt nine years ago when Mike and I lost a little girl through accidental poisoning. Life seems so fragile. I understand you have much to be optimistic about, and you must be grateful.

Best wishes to your whole family,

Lee McBride

*　　　*　　　*

M/Gen Carl-Gustaf Stahl
Defense Material Works
Stockholm, Sweden

May 6, 1981

Dear Judy and Mike,

You must know that both Margretta and I are deeply concerned about the terrible accident that happened to your son. If there is anything we could do to help you please let us know.

I am returning **The Third Wave,** *which I borrowed, from Judy, apologizing for having kept the book too long. But it was very interesting reading.*

All the best to you all.

Yours sincerely,
Carl-Gustaf Stahl

* * *

Sue Dunn
Atlanta, Georgia

May 6, 1981

Dear Judy and Mike,

Buz and I were shocked and desolated by the news of John's accident. After the initial blow, however, we were **grateful** *he is alive and making progress daily. I am sure your attitudes and fortitude are a great help to his spirits.*

What are his interests: reading matter, games, etc.? What could we send that would give him a lift? Does he have a favorite author, like Westerns, puzzles, etc.?

Please know how much we have you and him on our minds. Joanne, too, always. How can we be helpful?

With love to all,

Sue

* * *

Ellen Singer
Swarthmore College
Swarthmore, Pennsylvania

May 7, 1981

Dear John,

My Dad sent me a copy of the letter you sent them. I'm so glad to hear that you are in good spirits! It made me really happy to hear that. (So I decided to write on this bright stationary in this bright color.)

School is almost over. I can't believe it! I had my Physics exam yesterday and English this morning. Physics went really well, and I don't know how English went, but who cares now 'cause they're over!

Now I don't have another exam until Wednesday, so I blew off the whole afternoon. I sat outside and did nothing. After I'm done with exams Wednesday, I think I'll hang around here for a day—to pack, party, etc. Then I'm headed to D.C.

I've got a job for the summer doing research, but it's in Poolesville MD, so I still need to find a place to live for the summer. Poolesville's just a little too far to commute. Mom told me last night that David got the job in Texas. Do you think he'll turn into a real "southern boy" down there—boots, hat, chaw (yuk), the works? I guess we'll have to wait and see.

Well, I guess I'll close. I think I'll take a nap before dinner since I've only had about eight hours sleep in the last two days.

Hope everything keeps progressing well. And don't forget you're a "strapper," (Strapping, virile, young man, who's a ladies man)—that's what the guys I've been hanging around with lately are.

Always—take care.

Luv ya,
Ellen

*　　　*　　　*

Mrs. Joanne Golden
Montgomery, Alabama

May 8, 1981

Dear John,

We received a letter from your Mother today telling us of your progress. You have been in our thoughts and prayers everyday so we were happy and relieved to learn how you are doing. People you probably don't know but who know your parents have asked about you. You are being remembered by any number of people.

It is hot in Montgomery and tonight we turned the air conditioner on for the first time. I held out as long as I could. I am just trying to prepare myself for what Florida and Georgia will be like this summer.

Johnny hasn't been fishing in a couple weeks. He has been busy trying to finish his papers & book reports. He is so ready to get back to doing his thing and leave the paper writing to someone else for a while.

I am mailing via the pouch a package with a couple of paperbacks and a tape for you.

You are always in our thoughts.

Sincerely,
Joanne Golden

* * *

Suzy Hawley
Alexandria, Virginia

May 8, 1981

Dear Judy & Mike,

It was so good to talk to you two weeks ago. You sounded great which made me feel better. It's ridiculous that you have to buoy up the spirits of those outside your family! Joanne sounded neat too. We had a nice, little chat.

Loved your letter—and thanks for taking the time to write. I know you're **so** *busy right now....About my going to Sweden. I'd love to go—have wanted to ever since you got there. I would like to be able to offer some help and if I can, I'd love to visit this summer. If you decide it would be too much, let me know. Also, I don't think it'll be a problem to wait until Dave gets home. Those three always had special time without Mom and loved it (and I have too!). Dave is planning on camping during his 30 days before the Pentagon. (My Gawd, it is true! He's going to that place!). And I'd rather be in Sweden than camping! Anyway, it'll work out—but so frustrating that the mail to him and back is so awful. I want to know what he thinks. Got a letter Thursday dated April 10!!! May have to call his person at the Pentagon to relay messages.*

Most important! The letter from John was ***wonderful!*** *Such a super kid he is. I was terribly impressed that he was so open. Most impressive was his concern about you all. He's a bright, sensitive, gutsy kid—and I don't need to tell you, do I? John will be a great contributor!*

'Member Ty? Well, he turned out to be a she and just got spayed! She's trying to help me write this and we're both struggling!

Love,
Suzy

* * *

Lt. Col. John Golden
Maxwell AFB, Alabama

May 9, 1981

Dear Mike and Judy,

Joanne and I are both thinking of you and John. I wish we were closer so we could talk and drink a beer and throw rocks at the "vik" or something. Let us know what we can do from Montgomery. Please keep us posted on John's progress.

I've read Joanne's letter so I see that she has told you all of my news. Robie Hackworth is in apprenticeship for Dean. He told me he would like to have Mike here as head of National Security Affairs, once he's gained his position (that's Hackworth as Dean—pardon my pronouns). I report to McDill the first week in June to begin recurrency training. The ironic thing is this recurrency training will bring me up to my needed "gate" time. I was only one month short. Moody is overloaded with lieutenant colonels, so I'll be competing with the pack for a squadron. But that's all I ask for as I'm fairly strong operationally and I can get things done.

We miss you both. As Joanne said, you don't have to talk, but it's nice to be physically close to people you care about.

Love,
Johnny

*   *   *

Dan Singer
Washington, D.C.

May 10, 1981

Dear John,

A truly dreary rainy Sunday afternoon in Washington—chilly too, as if spring made a brief appearance last month to get the azaleas, tulips, dogwoods, etc. off and running for the current year, only to retire for sixty days until summer descends on us.

Stephanie is trying desperately to spur herself through her final boring, tedious days at NCS. If it weren't for the proms and parties and the return home of her siblings this week, I think she'd be a raving maniac by June 1 or so when school officially ends.

Dave will be the first home of the college generation, due to arrive Tuesday night to stay a few days and then off to Texas to make his first million hauling pipe on some oil derrick someplace.

Ellen is due back Thursday—she'll be looking for a place to live in Poolesville while she works at NIH animal experimentation facility—she's lined up a job with the world's greatest artificial inseminator.

Amy will be home next weekend and will go to work promptly with the Washington office of the Jerusalem Post, an English language daily published in Israel. She's **very** *excited about that.*

Steph has two weeks of pure play starting June 1 before leaving for six weeks in the French Alps polishing her French etc.

*Thanks much for your letter. (I know Maxine has already suggested that you take a course in spelling—***NOT** *taught by David.) Suzy Hawley keeps us posted on the details and I gather things are looking up. Our best for you.*

Love,
Dan

* * *

Mary Keating Russell
Santa Fe, New Mexico

May 11, 1981

Dear John,

I am very sorry that you have experienced such a tragic accident and I am writing to tell you that your Russell cousins wish you a rapid and successful recovery and full rehabilitation. In my work, I have made many friends who have met with accidents or war-related experiences resulting in severe injuries. One of my co-workers (confined to a wheelchair), a man in his mid-20's, has visited with me about the difficulties of physical rehabilitation and attitude adjustments that a person who has suffered an accident must undergo. I urge you to be aware that there will be really rough days, real down days, and that you should try to avail yourself of the best rehabilitation program available and identify individuals who share your experience, to talk to. If I can be of help, let me know.

Our best to the rest of the family and good luck to you.

Mary Russell

* * *

Mr. and Mrs. William Hamilton
Embassy of the United States
Stockholm, Sweden

May 12, 1981

Dear Judy and Mike,

We rejoice at each reported bit of progress and continue to admire the courage you two and Joanne, as well as John, display every day.

Jeanne and Bill

*　　*　　*

Mrs. Walter Burgess
Warren, Maine

May 12, 1981

Dear Great Grand Son:

A few lines to let you know I am thinking of you and ***thinking*** *of you! Wish all your USA folks could come in to see you. We are so glad to hear such a good report as to how you are getting along.*

I just can't realize what you are going through. I do hope the doctors are keeping you as comfortable as possible. It's a miracle what can be done now days in the medical line, so we all hope this terrible accident can be overcome, so your adjustment won't be too severe.

I have arthritis in my right arm and shoulder. I can't lift my arm up. I have to reach for things with my left hand. I can put my arm forward but not back. I tie my arm in front then pull it around back. It's very hard to cut meat or mash any food as I sit at the table. I am lucky to be as well as I am at 88 yrs. Do they have black flies in Sweden? They are **TERRIBLE** *here, the air is full of them, they go up sleeves, pant legs, down necks, into ears, hair, etc., bite leaves a black itching spot. They will be gone by June, then its mosquitoes.*

I do hope you keep gaining and can be moved nearer Stockholm before long. I have the oil heat on today; it's raining and too damp—no fire in the house. I'm listening to the Red Sox play ball. They are not doing very well, maybe I should take that back, as they are just 500, +13 and –13, were +8 and –13, have won the last 5 games. Four or five of their better players went to other clubs this season so I don't see how they can expect to do much. Keep up your courage.

Love to everybody,

Great Grandma Burgess

*　　*　　*

James P. Keating, Jr.
Neenah, Wisconsin

May 13, 1981

Dear John,

Thank you for your very bright and encouraging letter! John Patrick graduates from U. of Wisconsin next Saturday. We're going down for the ceremony, which starts of 9:30 am!!! They do it at that hour so the grads don't spend all day before graduation in the bistros, bars and evil saloons of Madison!!

He gets a BS in Civil Engineering, then heads out to Pasadena, CA in mid June for a job with a small engineering firm. Not too bad—they're starting him at $1700/mo. plus $200/mo. car allowance.

Your cousin Mike is planning on being with you and family in Sweden in June. I've tried to intercept him in Ireland so he writes first (or phones) so you and Mike Sr. and Judy know when he's coming. Hopefully, your recovery will be far enough along so you guys can do some touring, sailing, etc. together.

Jimmy is home from Ann Arbor, for the summer, working at the foundry. He's as chipper and outgoing as always, more so now that he's acquired a girl friend. I haven't met her but she's due here in two weeks, for a short visit.

Kelly is on a co-op work-study program at her college—working on a vegetable and herb farm on Nantucket Island. She was ready to quit last week, because they've got her housed in a drafty converted chicken coop, and paying her the queenly sum of $2.00/hour for 10 hours/day.

John, I'm really pleased about your outstanding progress! Keep your eyes on the future—we can learn from the past but we can't do one damn thing to change it!!

Love,

Pete

*　　*　　*

Ambassador Rodney Kennedy-Minott
Monterey, California

May 15, 1981

Dear Judy & Mike,

I just heard of the ghastly news concerning your son, John. Words are inadequate but sentiments are not. You two, John, your daughter, are all very much on Polly's and my minds and we extend out love, sympathy and compassion.

I hope John makes a good recovery and with parents such as yourselves, I know his postoperative therapy and subsequent adjustments will be positive ones.

Again—our love to you all—

Most respectfully,

Rodney & Polly

* * *

Col. and Mrs. Frederick Tillman
Griffiss AFB, New York

May 15, 1981

Dear Mike and Judy,

CeCe and I were shocked when we heard of John's accident. There is little that we can say that will help but we want you to know that we share your grief and are thinking of your family during this trying time. Of course, if there is anything that we can do to help in any way, please let us know. We hope that the rest of you are in good health and that John will recover soon and quickly adjust. Tell him we are thinking of him and praying for his recovery.

Fred & CeCe

*   *   *

Major Dave Hawley
American Embassy
Sana'a, Yemen Arab Republic

May 16, 1981

Dear Mike and Judy,

Hope everything is going relatively well in Stockholm. After failing to receive any mail from the US for more than 50 days, I called Suzy (yes, it is possible from sunny Sana'a). Everything was well, but she was quite shaken by John's accident, as am I. She had written about a month ago, asking me to write you, but the letter never arrived.

After the initial pain of the news, I realized he did not die and has the chance to lead a productive life. Suzy indicated his attitude was good. That seems a good sign. The loss was great, but not catastrophic, and we all hope for the best in his future. Any attempt to express my feelings would result in a page of platitudes, but please know my family and I share your pain.

. . .

Probably she's told you of her plan to visit you after I get back. Boys and I and Bobbie and his son plan to go on a camping trip—chance to commune with nature and all that.

During a recent visit to Colorado Springs, I spent a great evening with Patti and Chuck. She's still stunning and Chuck was in a quandary. He's now buying gold mines, but had some bad feelings about a deal with a good old boy in Atlanta and was about to fly there to untangle the mess.

What are your plans, i.e. when do you rotate? We'll see you during out-briefs.

Yours,
Dave

* * *

Jamie Sullivan
St. Albans School
Washington, D.C.

May 16, 1981

Dear Keats,

It's really hard to think of something to say to open up this letter. What can I say? You know that all your friends back here at school are behind you all the way and wish they were nearby to do anything they could possibly do for you. We're all fighting with you. I keep thinking of the blast, Warner, Stabes, and I had up at UNH with you back in the fall. I ended up not applying and John got rejected! Anyway, John's going to go to Boston University and Stabes is probably going also. I'm gonna go to Trinity in Connecticut. Ernie's going to Rollins and he's pretty psyched.

I suppose Ernie and Brian told you about the lacrosse team. They weren't playing as well as they should be for a while. Anyway, yesterday, they played St. Stephens and really got it together. At the end of the first quarter they were losing 5-1. That was when they had enough and got down to business. They beat St. Stephens 9-5! Brian never played so well; talk about hot! As usual Ernie played his heart out and knocked the stuffen out of St. Stephen's attack. Ernie's pretty damn proud to be wearing your number. He got your letter yesterday and it made him really glad that he'd heard from you.

John, we all love you and think about you all the time. We wish you could be back here now with us but we know that's impossible. Keep it up, have a good time when it's possible and remember we're all behind you. If you get a chance and want to, write back some time. Take it easy.

Jamie

*   *   *

Anne L. Reynolds
Waban, Massachusetts

May 17, 1981

Dear Mike and Judy,

Carolyn and Al just told us the terrible news about John. We are just shattered as we know you must be—and we want you to know how strongly we share your grief and rage—and wish to hell there were something we could do. If nothing else we wish we were close enough to come and offer what comfort we can. I **know** *that you will all come through this and that John will have a productive life. You are all too strong and too tough not to pick up the pieces and* *continue—but at the moment all that is nonsense—and you are simply going through sheer unadulterated hell. You two have borne so much in your years together. I am sure that this seems the last straw—certainly we all feel so frustrated and sick at what has happened. We cannot believe it.*

The older I get, the more I cannot accept the sheer craziness of life of which this is such a startling example. Gege and I just wish we were close enough to scream with you, hug you or get drunk with you—to do whatever it takes to get through this time.

We send you four all our love and support.

Much love,
Suki and Gege

* * *

Alfred B. Lane
Boxford, Massachusetts

May 18, 198

Dear John,

I'm confident this letter will find you greatly improved and more comfortable. No doubt, by the time this arrives you will be in Stockholm. To merely write to you seems such a nothing thing to do, but unfortunately, I can't think of a damned thing else I can do at the moment! Please let us know if there is anything we can do for you—anything we can mail to you or whatever.

Life in Mass. continues in turmoil. David has nine days of school left and by hook or by crook I guess he'll stagger across the finish line. This senioritis is a pain in the ass! Dave finds himself with a cash flow problem at the moment. He has bought another truck and now has two plus a snowplow! The plan is to sell the first one he bought plus the snowplow then he will use his 1972 Dodge Power Wagon four-wheel drive! (I guess its better than driving a motorcycle.) This is the type of truck he wanted, but couldn't find originally and he is really excited about it. He'll sure pay to ride around in it at 14 MPG.

Hey, don't know if we ever told you, Steve is a Cubemister! What's that, you ask? Remember the Cube of multi-colored squares that you had so much success matching up? Well, Steve finally managed to complete the task of solid colors on all six sides. I have long since given up as has the rest of the family. I think I'll take the damn thing up to Grandma Burgess and let her give it a try.

My first spring work trip to Maine is on the docket for this weekend. It's strange how everyone else is busy, so lucky me, I'll be going up alone. You can't imagine what its like to rototill Grandma's garden and then plant it as the blackflies invade your mouth, eyes, nose, ears and every area of visible skin. You know, maybe I'll skip the trip myself. The tree you and I started cutting up is as we left it and will no doubt remain that way for some time to come.

Not that I don't have anything else to do; I recently had ten cord of log-length wood deposited in the front yard. What a pile it is. We have managed to get it nearly all cut up and thanks to a splitter we have the wood nearly split as well. Next comes the task of stacking. Oh well, it'll be enough to keep us warm for two winters so plan to enjoy the warmth of a fire with us if not this fall surely next.

From the world of sports our greatest pleasure has been watching the Boston Celtics win the NBA Championship. I realize basketball is not your sport but nevertheless you would surely have enjoyed some of the playoff games. It was amazing to see a well-motivated team defeat a team, 76ers that had more talent.

I've rambled on here for too long and no doubt by now you're anxious for me to shut up so I will! Seriously though and before closing, I do hope your recovery will be speedy and all pain diminishes rapidly.

Best regards,
Al

*   *   *

Pat Wood
Littleton, Colorado

May 18, 1981

Dearest Judy and Mike,

You have constantly been in our thoughts and prayers ever since Patti called to tell us of John's accident. Until now, I've been unable to sit down and tell you how terribly concerned we have been for you and your family. It's just been so difficult for me to express in words how much we love and care for you all, and I just hope that my lack of communication hasn't marred your hopes of our deep concern for John.

We learned from Patti last evening that Bari had spoken with you, Judy, and that John was out of intensive care. We thank God for that and continue to pray for his recovery.

If there's ever a time you'd like just to talk, please call us collect. We feel so helpless being so far away, but all of us here want you to know that each of us is pulling for you, John and Joanne.

May God give you the strength that you need at this time, and the guidance to you all and your whole family.

Our love and concern to all of you,

Pat & Stu

*   *   *

Joyce Buni
Needham, Massachusetts

May 24, 1981

Dear Judy, Mike, John, and Joanne,

I am writing to all of you as I know that what happened to John has happened to all of you and I want you to know you all have my thoughts, prayers, love and support as you work your ways forward to new and viable lives.

This Christopher news note—I have valued their publications on all themes for 20 years—came the day Suki called me with the news of John's situation.

If I can be of service in any way please let us know.

Joyce

*   *   *

Col. (Ret) & Mrs. H. James Peck
Lago Vista, Texas

May 24, 1981

Dear John,

Here we are in Lago Vista, Texas and you are far away in Sweden, but we hope you can feel the shock we had when we got your Mom's letter telling us about your accident. Oh, John, we are so very sorry. My first words after reading her letter were, oh no not Baby John, because that is what we called you just after you were born.

We want you to come to Lago Vista. It is just about 30 miles north of Austin, TX, which is a terrific city. You might like to go to the University of Texas, but of course we will have to teach you how to talk Texan. We know a few phrases like, "Ya'll come back and see us here? or hear?" We are not sure how to spell it. Our house is right on the water here. We have a sailboat that sleeps two people and I remember that you sailed in Alabama. It is very rural here. We feed the deer every day and birds too. Also have a humming bird in residence. So cute.

Pam and her husband live in Reston and they are expecting their first baby the end of June this year. Bill is studying to be an architect and Pam works for a newspaper. She majored in photography but is in advertising right now and likes it.

Golly, I have so many questions to ask you. When did you graduate from high school? How tall are you now? Have a special girl friend? See, old aunts want to make sure these girls are treating you right.

John, we will pray for you every day for a speedy recovery and convalescence. Your Mom said you might get home next month. I'm not sure when you will receive this. Hopefully soon. Take care, love ya.

Love,
Aunt Nita & Uncle Jim

* * *

St. Albans School
Mount St. Alban
Washington, D.C.

Headmaster's Study

May 26, 1981

Dear John:

I will be eager to know how your most recent operation came out. I do hope it went well.

It is hard to believe that we are closing in on graduation, but indeed, we are. With a victory over Georgetown Prep, the baseball team won the ICA title and thereby settled the Founder's Cup on St. Albans for the fourth straight year. Lacrosse ended the year with a ten and two record. In quite a few of those games, they came from way behind to win. Next year we are just going to play the last half of each game!

We've had the usual tears and cheers over college, but now the dust is settling and most people have the next few years planned. Continued best wishes to you.

Sincerely yours,
Mark H. Mullin
Headmaster

* * *

James P. Keating, Jr.
Neenah, Wisconsin

May 27, 1981

Dear Keatings—all—

We received Judy's letter a couple of weeks ago. You'd written it May 8, and apparently had someone hand-carry it to New York, where it was posted on May 11.

Your news continues to be **most** *encouraging. My respect for the Swedish physicians and the British hypnotist is considerable, but then they've got a* **tough** *and highly motivated young man to work with!!*

Michael Thomas, the world traveler, is now in Scotland staying with Kathy Keating Wilson's brother, Sam. Mike had his money, passport, & Visa card stolen in Dublin. He was "lulled into complacency" as he puts it, by the charm of Ireland—neglected to bring his valuables with him when he went to take a shower—and everything was gone when he returned. The Embassy people were very responsive, and he had money and a new passport in a matter of hours.

He's looking forward to visiting you in Stockholm, communicating with John—(Mike lost the ends of two fingers in an accident at the foundry last summer), so he can share, in a small degree, John's injury.

John Patrick graduated from Wisconsin a week ago, BS in Civil Engr. He bought a '79 Chevy and after several friends' weddings in early June and late May, leaves for Pasadena, Cal. where he's got a job with a small Engineering firm.

Keep up the great progress, **all** *of you. The nice thing about being a part of a super family is we can share our triumphs & travails alike!*

Love,
Pete

* * *

Stephanie Singer
Washington, D.C.

May 29, 1981

Dear John,

Thanks for your well-timed letter! I just had my last exam this morning. I still have a Brown math-take-home that's due Monday, though...

By the way, did you hear from Joanna, the girl who lived next door to us last summer? She said she wrote you. I wish I could send you something to **really** *cheer you up, maybe a can of electric pink paint to splatter randomly on the monotonous walls. Or you could spill it on your least favorite nurse.*

This week was rough because my grandmother died. We went up to New York Tuesday for the funeral. I'm a little worried about my Mom (it's her mother) because she's kept cool so far but I know it's going to hit her sometime.

That's great that you're standing and even mobile! I don't know why but I've had some silly idea of you sitting in a hospital bed, in traction, swathed with bandages, with a hole for your nose, **maybe**. *It's good to find out you're not mummified.*

I leave for France on the 15th of June. I've never been before. I'll be living with a French family. It should be a blast.

The Singer household is a little hairy with everyone home—when Amy and David get together, I head for the nearest fall-out shelter.

To relieve the boredom—you might get yourself a Rubik's cube. I have one, but every time I get anywhere near figuring it out Dave grabs it and ruins **everything!**

Love,
Steph

*   *   *

Col. & Mrs. P.K. Crawley
American Embassy
Cairo, Egypt

May, 1981

Dear All,

Many thanks for your note and for keeping us informed on John's progress. Gee, that young man is really put together with good stuff to have come through his experience. The Keating Family has had our emotional and spiritual support.

This assignment has been a can of worms since day one. What we did to deserve this place, I'm not sure. We keep telling ourselves, we will overcome, ha! But I'm sinking! We were sitting some rows back of Sadat on the fateful day. What an emotional and frightful experience. Had all the hand grenades exploded, the death and injury total would have been much greater. The scene is well imprinted and not a day passes that it isn't relived. Life here is very difficult and this country defies description.

I miss Fru Sven so much. If you meet her on her terms she will produce good dinners for you and she is such a dear. I think of her so often and long to have her here.

Olof & Catherine Wallander visited us last month and we had a delightful time. I plan to return to Florida in late January and "try to put myself together" and visit ailing parents and get some work completed for them.

Dearest love to John, Joanne and all. Come to Egypt. It defies description. Must see to believe.

Best wishes for a splendid New Year!

Fondly,
Vivian Faye & PK

* * *

Susan Lane
Boxford, Massachusetts

May, 1981

Dear John,

Hello! How are you coming along? I hope you're making progress and emotionally okay. I guess I can have no conception of what you're going through, but I've been thinking a lot about you and I wish I could see you. Well, I guess you can live without my wise cracks for just a little longer. I bet you're upset about that!!!

Nothing much is going on around here. Don't even mention school!! Yuek, I'm so bored with it, but that's the breaks I guess. It's been starting to get warm here (thank God.) I really love the hot sun and I can't wait for summer.

Oh yeah, I've been mystifying all the kids I baby-sit with your wonderful card tricks. Especially the one when you slip the card from the bottom and guess it without looking at it. (I'm so tricky.) I still think you should have revealed the secrets to your other ones!!

So, what's Animal up to? Notice how I capitalized his name!! We haven't had any rowdie sock fights recently. Too bad. I, the lazy slob, am not working this summer. No comments! I know I should. I'll do some babysitting. It's pretty hard to find work when you go away for three weeks though (Maine). Oh, Maine, that should be exciting. I don't know if I can hack it for three weeks. It's fun and everything, but after about one week of not seeing anyone under the age of 65, it gets to you a little. Well, listen, take care of yourself. Hello to Joanne!!

Love,
Susan

* * *

Ingrid S. Beach
Washington, D.C.

June 1, 1981

Dear Judy and Mike,

Ned and I have so often had you in our thoughts for many weeks, and finally I'm sitting down to tell you of our profound sympathy over the accident that has befallen your John. At the same time, however, we rejoice over the fact that he has survived a voltage, which could have been fatal.

Dave Moss has kept us up on developments and from Maggie Feller, we've had our latest report. Both of them tell us that John has a superb morale. This strength of his own combined with the wonderful parental support he's getting from you, and the excellent hospital care he's undoubtedly receiving, will I'm sure lead to a recovery that will leave John handicapped but in other respects his usual self.

If John is at all interested in studying Swedish while he's convalescing, let us know and we'll mail you a complete sample copy of our soon-to-be-published book, plus it's almost completed tapes. This book is especially directed towards a self-study pupil (although for classroom use also) with easy to understand grammatical explanations **in English** *and good self-study exercises.*

Please let us do anything else you can think of within our power. Has John read **all** *of Ned's books? Otherwise we'll send the missing ones.*

Do make sure that **you** *also take care of* **yourselves** *after the ordeal you* **too** *have lived through. Hans Neij says that you are so highly thought of in the Swedish community.*

Give John our most heartfelt wishes for a good recovery, to your sweet daughter a warm hug, and to you, dear friends our deep love,

Ingrid and Ned

* * *

Sandra Lane
Rosendale, New York

June 1, 1981

Dear John,

We were all so glad to hear from you. Thanks very much for the letter. You sounded in very good spirits in your letter and we were thrilled to hear that you are surprising the doctors with your fantastic recovery. That sounds like a very good sign. We all sure hope your progress continues that way until you're back to "full strength." Hope all the operations are over now and that the phantom pains and nightmares have subsided.

Everything is going along about the same here. Jack is working very hard at his new job and it will be very different for him not having the entire summer off. The kids are studying for final exams now—their last day of school is June 17th.

My parents were just here for a week and we all had a nice visit. We planted just a few things in a tiny garden plot. Mainly we would like a few fresh tomatoes and cukes. We are planning a couple of quick trips to Maine this summer. Jack has one week in July and one in August. Brian has to look around town for a job as he just bought Alan's trail bike for $600 and he only had $200—so he's missing a few bucks!!

When you feel in the mood, drop a line and let us know how you're doing.

Love and all our best wishes,

Sandra, Jack, Alan, & Brian

* * *

Gail and Tony Cashen
Ghent, New York

June 3, 1981

Dear Judy and Mike and John and Joanne,

I was terribly saddened to hear of John's accident and all the struggle he has had since then. Of course, that feeling was soon overtaken with a great sense of relief that he has the toughness and determination to do so well. From your letter, I conclude that he has just had another in the series of operations and I certainly hope that one went well. I know you will be relieved when he can begin spending some time at home and perhaps fatten him up a little.

The Keatings have always been determined people and I am sure your support is what has made it possible for him to keep plugging away. No one can imagine the grief that this has been for you all. Please send him our love. I remember what a tough kid he was and I know he will make it. I am also so very glad he is going to pull through.

After four years of trying to keep the lumber business in Tupper Lake afloat, Tony finally liquidated it and has assumed the presidency of Flanagan and Webster, a small executive recruiting firm in the city. He likes the work and is good at it and seems resigned to working for someone else again, although this is a pretty independent kind of business—each one pretty much does his own thing.

I am still teaching at the College of New Rochelle, have finished the doctorate and have been taking a course in computer science this past semester, which I found very interesting.

Susan was graduated in June from St. John's College in Santa Fe, New Mexico and is now living and working in Ann Arbor, Michigan. Harper spent a social year at State University College in Potsdam, has now taken two years off, and has made application to return. I hope he applies himself this time, now that he has some better notion of what the world is like if you don't have a college degree or a good trade (poor). Mike has been a good student and will be going to Cornell in the fall. Tony's eldest daughter has taken time off after finishing two years at the University of Colorado, his second daughter is going to Switzerland on an exchange program, and his third daughter is still in high school.

Please let me know if there is anything I can do for you or, particularly, for John. We are very near the city, as you remember, and it would be easy for me to make any contact, which might be helpful, or to send anything. I would like to contribute to keeping his spirits up if there is anything I could do.

We are looking forward to seeing you next summer. Do you have any idea where you might be stationed? You have an open welcome here, of course, for as long as might be convenient. Thanks for letting me know how things are. Please let me know what we can do.

Love,
Gail & Tony

* * *

Col. & Mrs. Giles Harlow
Vance AFB, Oklahoma

June 3, 1981

Dear Mike & Judy,

Gail called me yesterday—from New York and in the middle of the day—and of course I knew instantly something was wrong. She'd just gotten your letter and was very shaken—said she'd wandered around her house for about an hour feeling sick before she'd called. We are all terribly distressed and upset to learn the news about John's accident and its aftermath. I just can't imagine what you all have gone through, you've certainly had many more than your share of trouble—it all seems terribly unfair and tragic to us. We're very thankful that John has survived and are remembering him and you all in our prayers but we're still just terribly sorry. I wish there were something we could do for you—we feel so helpless.

Life goes on here at Vance—we graduate about 50 new pilots every six weeks and are enjoying our tour here very much. Chip graduated from Clemson last month and starts pilot training at Reese on October 6—wonder if he'll land in Mike's field! He'd put Vance second on his list of choices because he was afraid we'd still be here. He and Doug are back up in Alaska working for the same guy they did last summer—they love it up there—says it's like Colorado without the man-made scars. Doug's still at U. of Texas, hanging on by his fingernails in M.E.*—he may be there forever. Bitsy starts U. of Colorado in August—She's home for the summer and life guarding at the Base pools. And Sally's still down in Austin swimming but will be home in August.*

No word on a future assignment for us—I've started a graduate course in political science that OSU offers here on Base (have 12 hours now & am taking two courses this summer) and am hoping we'll be here long enough for me to get at least within a thesis of the degree. Giles takes shameful advantage of his position and flies as much as possible—at least three times a week, sometimes more. No general's on base—he's the big cheese and loves every minute of it. We're in for a comedown! And with my parking places right smack in front of the commissary and BX, all my career goals have been met.

Please give John our love and tell him we're pulling for him. Thank God you all are so solid—eventually things will work out but I must admit we find it all hard to understand and accept sometimes.

Love,
Ann

* * *

Bernice Williams
Neenah, Wisconsin

June 4, 1981

Dear Mike and Judy,

So glad to hear from you and happy to hear that John is making progress. How wonderful that the hypnotism worked. We think of you every day, and our hopes and love go out to you all. We keep Karen and Tom and John and Jan informed of any news from you.

You probably know that Lyal has his surgery on his left eye and so far, he's progressing well, he can now see to read, and do most of his bookwork etc. Still can't drive, and must not lift or bend way over—so, of course, can't play golf—he's hoping to be able to swing a club by the end of the summer. I'm still running on the golf course and keeping up my other activities, and of course, chauffeuring Lyal. So keep very busy.

Andrew (No. 4 boy) graduates from high school Sunday, so we'll spend the day in Niagara. Though he's not been officially notified, the coach at the Merchant Marine Academy called and said he's been accepted. We all hope so 'cause that's what he wants, architecture is his field.

Do hope John is out of intensive care now. I suppose tragedy has to be accepted and coped with but our hearts ache for all of you.

Love,

Bernice

* * *

B/Gen & Mrs. W.P. Bowden
Bolling AFB, D.C.

June 10, 1981

Dear Mike and Judy,

My heart goes out to you when I think of all you've gone through these past few months—I only wish we had been there to provide moral and emotional support. We pray that John will continue to recover as expected and that his courage and strength remain strong! I am so glad you found good medical care there and agree it was good the four of you could be together instead of leaving John at Brooke. I know the State Department and Embassy folks are helpful but if there's ***anything*** *we can do from this end, especially now that we are in D.C., don't hesitate to call.*

We arrived here and moved in April 1. (It wasn't an April Fool's joke—this is the one place I never was thrilled about returning to but no one ever asked us!) Bill's the Deputy Director Logistics Plans & Programs (LEX). He likes it here—I prefer a slower, quieter pace. The traffic has increased tremendously since we left in '72.

We like these quarters (new ones). They are large and the only thing we don't have is big trees. Am about used to National Airport noise! Andy is home for the summer; he really likes Oklahoma State. Marjorie is attending St. Mary's Academy in Alexandria. She doesn't like going to school without boys, but she's managing! She's in Oklahoma now for two weeks visiting all her friends back there—she really left "roots" there and plans to go to Oklahoma State next year!

Enough of us—take care and a hug to y'all and especially to John. Keep us posted!

Love always,
Bill & Isobel

* * *

Mrs. Walter Burgess
Warren, Maine

June 13, 1981

Dear Grandchildren,

This letter is especially to congratulate Joanne on her achievement to graduate and to wish Judith a nice birthday, July 2nd. I am putting in a check. Please give Joanne $15.00 as a graduation gift, she has done so well. The other $5.00 is a birthday gift for Judith.

I am of course thinking of John many times every day. What a siege he is going through. We can't realize it, to say we are sorry doesn't do much good. I do hope he can be moved nearer to home soon.

I know it is hard for all of you, Mike and Judith and Joanne. I pray God to give John strength and courage for all he is going through.

Sadie is planning to go to Littleton, NH June 23 to an Eastern Star thing to honor her. I do hope she has a nice trip and gets back safely. She asked Gladys Cramer to go with her but Gladys isn't going.

Soon you folks will be on your last year in Sweden. I do hope you have less trouble. How lucky we don't know what is ahead. Wish we could do more to help you. I can't put cards in this kind of letter but I do congratulate Joanne so very much on her graduation, and try to have a nice Birthday, Judith.

Do you remember Walter had a brother Charlie Burgess; he died about two years before Walter. His widow Olive died June 5, was with her daughter Eve Burgess Newell of Florida. Services last Tuesday in Union. Take care the best you can, love to you all. Think of you so many times each day. Wish I could help you.

Love to all,
Grandma Burgess

*   *   *

Justin Walker
Washington, D.C.

June 22, 1981

Dear Johnny,

How ya doing, buddy boy? Your letter was great and I'm glad to hear you're in good spirits. Right now it's a Monday afternoon in the big city and I got off work early. You see, I'm driving a delivery truck for a florist. I deliver flowers, and sometimes there aren't too many deliveries to make, like today.

Oh yeah, just about everyone I talked to at these graduation parties asked about you, and I sort of told them that you were doing well and that it would be real cool if they wrote you. Of course, most of them were bossy women, but what else would you expect.

Heck, I heard Davey, Bill, and Carl all gave you a telephone call a while back, sorry I missed it but somewhere along the way there was a "Communication Breakdown" (Led Zep) between Dave and myself. They said it was great talking to you.

I just went in and grabbed a frosty cold Budweiser and I think I'll chug it down for you, O.K.? Here goes....Buurrrpppp!!!!! Whew, that sure hits the spot.

My Mom just got home and she says hello and sends her love. Well listen brother, you know how it gets in the summer time; things get slow and news is scarce—so I'd truly appreciate a fine, long letter from ya telling about everything and anything. I'd like to know how you're feeling, because you're one of my best friends and I care about you. So I'll be waiting to hear from you and till then take care of yourself and remember

SEE IT ALL!!

Love,
Jud

*   *   *

BG & Mrs. H.P. Houser, III
7th USA Tng. Comd. USAREUR
APO New York 09114

June 27, 1981

Dear Judy and Mike,

Just received a letter from Ann Harlow telling me of your son's accident. I sent the letter on to Mom and Dad as I know they too would want to know. Parks and I are just so saddened to hear of this tragedy. I'm sure it's been quite an ordeal to watch this in your beloved son. Just praying that God is surrounding you with His love and providing you strength and courage to face each day. Surely He is the only One who truly understands our every thought and emotion and can fortify us. He promised in His word not to give us more that we can bear, but will give us His grace. Have any of you read the story of Joni Erickson? Perhaps it would be of some comfort. Autobiography of a young girl, paraplegic.

Please call on us if there is anything at all we can do. You are in our prayers.

Love,
Sue

*　　　*　　　*

Sylvia Clements
Vienna, Virginia

June 29, 1981

Dear John,

Many who knew you and your family in Montgomery keep you in their thoughts and prayers daily and send love across the miles to you for a speedy recovery.

With affection,

Sylvia Clements

Especially for you

WITH WARMEST THOUGHTS

Hope it will make
the day brighter,
perhaps a bit cheerier, too
To know that someone
is thinking
so often, so fondly of you!

* * *

Col. (Ret.) and Mrs. Roy Doran
Austin, Texas

June 29, 1981

Dear Judy and Mike,

We just received word about John from Ann Harlow via Sue and Parks. We were most distressed to hear of John's accident. Things like this are hard to understand but I know from experience that if we put our trust in the Lord at times like this it somewhat eases the pain. I can well remember John as a little tyke and we hope and pray that he will be able to adjust to his handicap.

We also heard from Ann that Joanne is moving along. She was such a sweet thing as a little girl and I am sure she still is as she has blossomed into a young lady.

Tell John to keep his chin up just as his granddad would have done.

Our love to you both,

Roy

Dear Ones,

What sad news to receive. Our prayers are with you all. Wish we could be of some help to all of you. There is so much to be done daily in new fields of handling such problems as John's.

God bless all of you.

Love,
Lucile

*   *   *

Susan Lane
Boxford, Massachusetts

June 30, 1981

Dear John,

Hello! How are you doing? Well, I hope. All's fine here. Being out of school is great. It was really nice to get your letter and hear how you're doing.

I have to apologize for my writing though because once I'm out of school I don't really care. As you'll soon figure out, I'm not coordinated either. I can't handle this writing without lines.

Life in Boxford remains motionless. I've been having a good summer though. The normal pattern includes making money babysitting and then spending money shopping and going out. The only way to go, right!! Myself and two friends rode our bikes 17 miles to the beach today. That was great, but when we got there it was cold and cloudy. We didn't stay long. So all I have to show for that is sore legs and sandy toes. No tan and we didn't even go in the water. What a waste!! My tan definitely needs help.

We leave for Maine Friday, June 3. I haven't thought about that much yet. I guess it'll be okay. David's coming home on the 14th for a concert. Mom and I are coming back on the 16th. I have to start work the next day. I'm working at a camp nearby that is for retarded and handicapped kids. I'm going to be a swim-aid mostly I think. That will be something new and I'm really looking forward to it. I'm also going to be playing softball some nights, so with that and babysitting, I'll have enough to do.

What I really need though is my license. I guess I'll get around to that someday. Love to Joanne and your parents. Take care!

Lots of love,
Susan

*　　*　　*

Col. (Ret) and Mrs. Robert Burman
Alexandria, Virginia

June 30, 1981

Dear Judy & Mike,

Bob and I just returned from a month's vacation in California and Arizona—came home to read your sad news about John's experience. We can truly appreciate the shock and numb feeling you must have felt for some time. Praise God he is alive and also that you do have such great support from all of those close who care. I do hope that John continues to get the support that he alone will need, most surely as time goes on from all his own friends. You will all be and are in our hearts and prayers. You are such a lovely family and I know you are being loved well and supported by many, many people. You give so much, so now it is your turn to receive some of that giving from those who care. That's what life is all about and those of us who hopefully know what community means can receive the strength we need in the bad times as well as the good times.

Am happy to know all else is going smoothly for you. We wish it had been in the cards for us to come to Sweden but sometimes there are other plans made for us. Wish I could have seen Britt and Andres also, but Bob had a great visit.

Will get a longer letter off as soon as grandchildren leave. I now feel my 60 years—can't keep running every day but love it.

Fondly,
Barbara & Bob

* * *

St. Albans School
Mount St. Alban
Washington, D.C.

Headmaster's Study

July 10, 1981

Dear John:

Dave Singer told me that you had been able to get out of the hospital and go home for a few days. That is wonderful! He is certainly looking forward to visiting you this summer, and I am looking forward to hearing his report of how you are doing.

Summer has arrived in Washington with its usual heat and humidity, but we had a terribly wet Fourth, so all those who headed for the beaches stayed inside to play poker. I was away from school for a while attending Day School for Headmasters' meeting in Atlanta. The meeting was good, but I was a little disappointed in Atlanta. I had always heard what a great city it was. I guess there are not many U.S. cities that are as beautiful as Washington.

I do hope that you continue to make progress. It is great news for all of us when we hear from you.

Sincerely yours,

Mark H. Mullin
Headmaster

* * *

Mrs. Maloney
Washington, D.C.

July 1981

Dear John,

You must know we've all been thinking about you—praying for you and aching in our hearts and souls for all you've gone through. When the reports finally started coming in that you were feeling better, doing better, flirting with nurses and all that nonsense, only then did we feel a little better ourselves. I know there certainly isn't anything I can say in this letter that you don't already know about how much we all **care** *and please know how very much you've been in out thoughts. Summer goes so fast. Michael is in Nantucket "working" and living with friends of ours, Kathleen is doing some intern work for a fellow who produces 20/20 (TV Documentary-type program), Paul is at Hilton Head Island working at his father's property down there, clearing land (with T. Walker & M. Collins), Anne is taking a Pre Calculus course (Mr. Brown) at STA and taking Driver's Education (Oh God, not another DRIVER in the family!!), Patrick is at camp in Virginia for six weeks and loving it. So because Father Maloney is gone all week usually, there are nothing but females around the household this summer (Fewer problems!)*

We may get to Nantucket in August—although in shifts. Kath doesn't finish her French course at Georgetown University until middle of August—Jinny will come back from California then to see us at Nantucket—about that time Paul will have to be back in D.C. for football practice—our last summer for **that** *and so on—*

I'm taking a French course myself and loving it although there is never enough time to practice. Since Kath will be studying at the Sorborne next year, I thought it would be nice to be able to speak the language when I go see her in Paree!!

Dean Stambaugh is retiring at the end of the next school year, which really surprises me—somehow I thought he'd be there til he died. We're having a big sort of retrospective around Christmas time with lots of old—old, old—student's works included. I'm on the "planning committee" which I thought would be fun since I get such a kick out of that lovely old man.

Please give your whole family our love, best wishes and assurance that you all are in our thoughts.

Hoping to see you soon, John dear,

I remain, fondly,

OLD LADY MALONEY

*　　　*　　　*

Anne Maloney
Washington, D.C.

July 25, 1981

Well John,

I finally set my ink to paper. When David said he was leaving DC soon, I decided that it was about time to write (since I'd save stamps by giving the letter to him!!) No, I can't say that I've been busy because I really haven't been. However, I can say that I'm lazy, cuz I have been.

The only **constructive** *activity I'm partaking in is a Pre Calculus course at STA. My teacher is Mr. Brown and I arise at 7:30 each morning to be at class at 8:00 (until 10:00). My poor Math course has been neglected though as I have yet to complete one assignment. I am passing though I started off planning to do my work daily, but for the first two weeks of class, Earnesto got me into the habit of pretending to do my homework and then going out* *at exactly 10:00 pm every night. So, I have been unable to break my routine of placing Math at the bottom of my list of priorities.*

Right now Ernie is at home in Florida but he may come back up ***very soon****. He told me to say "Hi" if I wrote to you—Ernie says "Hi" and Brian S. says, "Keats man, what's up?" and they both say, "Take it easy!"*

Last week I went to STA vs. Landon summer lacrosse game. STA was ***way*** *behind but they caught up and won. Good game. Stabes was quite good with 2 assists and two goals. Last spring season his good luck charm was a dark green bandana about the color of this pen. I don't know if you remember, but last Thanksgiving when we went to* **Ireland's Four Provinces,** *you wore it (I lent to you.) and he took it and put it on. Well, we made a deal that he could keep it until the end of last season as long as he wore it every game. So he did and by graduation, it meant so much to him that I gave it to him for a graduation present. Anyway he had it at the game last weekend and it paid off.*

Oh, the other day I was walking home from STA when some man drove up behind me and I heard a male voice say, "Hey, cutie," I next saw that it was this scruffy-looking man and thought it was just some pusher or something, but soon found out otherwise—it was Jud in his flower delivery truck. I couldn't stop laughing as I rode home in the fragrant thing. He seems to be having a good summer but wants to get away from D.C. SO DO I! Mike is up at Nantucket with Melissa. He's working as a landscaper and making good money (but has been spending a lot) that goes without saying. Justin wants to go visit him. Our family is going up in 1½ weeks for a month so he might be able to.

I got my license a while ago, so will be able to drive around up there. Should be fun. I have to go turn over my Santana record because it's over on this side. (I saw Carlos in concert a few weeks ago and he was great—five encores!! Also saw Al Jarrean two nights ago and he was excellent too.)

So now I feel better that I've filled you in on my activities and I wish you'd write back soon. I hear that you're doing well and getting around fine and all that makes me happy. Still it would make my day if I were to hear from you. TAKE CARE. Miss ya,

Love,
Killer

* * *

Mrs. Walter Burgess
Warren, Maine

July 27, 1981

Dear Great Grand Son:

I do hope you receive this in time for your birthday. I did not realize Aug. 10 was so near. Nana received Joanne's letter. We are all so glad to know you are able to be home. I know being home will add to your Happy Birthday. We all do hope this coming New Year will be better in every way for you.

We can't realize what you have gone through. You have shown such courage; wish we could help you more. Thank you **so** *much for the lovely picture I was so pleased with it and with Judith's card telling how you all are. Alfred (2 weeks) and Jack (1 week) and families have been in Maine for their vacation. Jack comes again in August (week of 10th); they all read the card Judith sent and saw your picture.*

*We are so glad to know you are coming along so well. Sadie will probably be writing to you and telling you about things she is having done on the house at West Rockport. She has had sadness—her Buttercup got killed, supposed hit by a car—she has a new 6-weeks old kitten—***cute***. Black and white female—slick hair marked so even—black coal bonnet, face, tail and* *white throat, chest, paws. "Puffy!" She is so fat like a puffball. Goes for first distemper shot today.*

I do hope this year will go fast and you folks will be back in the USA by this time in 1982 AND no more accidents. Big wedding Wednesday. I will have to get up early to watch on TV. Prince Charles and Lady Diana.

I must close its almost mail time and not much more room. Do have as happy a Birthday as possible. ***Keep*** *gaining—we all think of all of you. Everyone take care.*

Much love,
Great Grandma Burgess

*　　　*　　　*

Susan Lane
Boxford, Massachusetts

July 27, 1981

Dear John,

Hi! What have you been up to? Bet home is great. Hope you're doing well.

Life here is good. I work about a half-day and then softball at night. Work's okay. Although one of the kids got lost yesterday. We found him a couple of miles down the road in a police car. Strange job!! We took the kids to Salisbury Beach last week and that was fun.

As for softball, we won't discuss it. It's too depressing. I can't even use the adjectives to describe how well I play in case your parents read this. To make life better he (coach) has put me at catcher. I hate it and I don't play well at all. Oh well…

Sorry I didn't type it as Stephen did. I'm sure you can't read this, but with typing I can never think of anything to say. Not that this is much better, but…

I went camping with a friend last weekend. It was a nice place on the ocean in Maine. We did have a rather interesting experience. On Saturday, we went hiking on the trails. After about a half-hour, we came to a nice little secluded beach. We and a few others were there swimming, sunning, and hacking around. Though some of us were getting more sun than others. About six people who all came separately, thought it was a great beach for sun bathing without a bathing suit. Well I'm sure some of them were very sore that night. It was quite a shock to be at a beach with naked people, but we decided not to join them. Too bad!! I hope you're having a better time and making good progress. Have a good day. Smile for me!!

Love,
Sue

* * *

Stephen Lane
Boxford, Massachusetts

July 29, 1981

Dear John,

We are very glad you are home. Joanne wrote us a letter and told us you went home. How do you like the "Rubic's Cube" we sent you? A month or so ago, I finished the hole (sic) thing. After I finished it I figured out how to take it apart and then put it together the write (sic) way, but it was harder to put it together than I thought.

A week ago we were on vacation, and I tried water-skiing. I got up! On the last weekend of our vacation, just my father and I stayed so their (sic) weren't enough people for me to water-ski, but one day Nana came over and she spotted for me.

Love,
Stephen

Dear John,

We were so pleased to receive a letter from you. It meant a great deal to us. Excuse our sporadic correspondence and this mixed up letter (Everyone wants to get their say in, I guess.) Home must be extra special at this time having been deprived of your privacy and all the goodies it can provide. Hope all is going well and you are continuing to be able to chart progress.

Love to all,

Aunt Carolyn & Uncle Al

*　　　*　　　*

Brian Stableford
Washington, DC

August 14, 1981

Dear Keats,

What's up man? So, how have you been? Cool! Anyway I bet you never thought to hear from me, huh? So, I've just been hanging out here in D.C.

all summer pretty beat. Worked for a while as an office clerk. I couldn't stand it! Played summer lacrosse. Got messed up. A lot! Not playin lacrosse though. Anyway you know me.

Earnesto was up here with me these last twelve days; it was cool. Now he's back down in Florida getting ready for soccer at Rollins. Boley has been hanging out too. He made $6000 this summer out in Arizona. He bought a new car and a great stereo for it. So, everyone has been pretty cool. I'm getting ready for college—I can hardly wait. I'm going to Boston University. It oughta be cool. I think Kerns is going too. Anyway, I'm going to play lacrosse for them. I've been offered a scholarship for my sophomore year. I'm psyched. Who else have you heard from? Take care.

Love you,
Stabes

* * *

Stephanie Singer
Washington, DC

August 16, 1981

Dear Johnny,

I've got the alarm set for 8:00 tomorrow morning but I'm just too wound up to sleep. Dad and I just got back from Curacao today. (I sent you a postcard—please disregard my snide remarks about D.C.—I was just trying to say how much I liked Paris.) I was so glad to be home. On the way back from the airport, Mom told me that Big Ed had left his bass and amp here for me to try out while he went to Canada for a week. I was so excited I just smiled and smiled, non-stop. I smiled when I plugged it in and smiled when I tried (with little success) to play and I smiled as I unpacked, just thinking about the bass. In fact, I didn't stop smiling until, when I took a break to practice my 'cello, my new bow broke. It broke! It snapped at the tip. Well, that brought me down quickly. But then Katherine came by, laden with Beatles albums, and I was glad to see her again, and best of all, Dave came home tonight. We had dinner at about 11:00 pm with all of us (minus Ellen, who's at the beach), Dave's roommate Israel and his girl-friend, Wiggy and Eleanor, and Amy's boyfriend. It was great fun and I was so happy to be home, I just laughed and laughed and smiled and smiled, almost to the point of embarrassment. That was a while ago, but my adrenaline is still running.

I leave for school the 28th—I wish I had a little more time to be in D.C. – isn't it funny how good friends and things to do, places to go, all come together and pile up triumphantly just as one is about to leave. But I am looking forward to meeting my roommates.

Dave said you're taking Swedish lessons!! Ja, Ja, gud! Or however you say it.

What else is new? You ask. Well, I've completed my nerdly image by getting a subscription to Scientific American. I'm in the middle of a **very** *long,* **very** *long French novel. The evening is actually* **cool** *here in D.C.! I have a wonderful little crush on a guy named Paul who is lead singer in Big Ed's band and who is the ultimate in teenage rock-band COOL. Oh, and Mom bought me sheets and a comforter for school—I really don't like the pattern or the colors, but I won't let her know. Actually, it's not that important—I shut my eyes when I sleep anyway.*

Love,
Steph

*   *   *

Jeff Steinbach
Harvard University
Cambridge, Massachusetts

August 26, 1981

Dear John,

I just received a copy of the St. Albans bulletin, and realized as I read through our class notes that I still hadn't written to say how relieved and happy I was to hear of your speedy recovery and of Dave's trip to visit you this summer.

I'm sure Dave and Co. have kept you busy—how are the Swedish women and the Swedish bars anyway? I know there has to be some incentive to recover and get back into the scene!!

In case Dave hasn't' told you. I really didn't like Swarthmore. Anyway, Nassi Samiy and I are both transferring to Harvard and will be sharing an apartment in Cambridge fairly close to the center of campus. I am psyched since there are quite a few people from our class in the Boston area. The idea of having our own apartment ain't bad either.

By the time you get this I'll already be up in Boston. But I don't actually start until the 21st of September. If you get a chance, drop me a line. I'd like to hear about Dave's visit since it sounded like it was going to be some kind of trip.

Best wishes,
Jeff

* * *

Stephanie Singer
Yale University
New Haven, Connecticut

September 4, 1981

Johnny,

I am settling in here at Yale. My schedule is pretty much set—Math Physics, Music, and French. I like all my courses so the work (lots of it) shouldn't be too much trouble.

This weekend is filled with auditions of all sorts. Auditions for plays, for various choruses and for the Yale Symphony. Surprisingly, my first priority is the symphony. In fact, I've suddenly gotten a lot more serious about the 'cello and about music in general. A lot of it comes from hanging around so much with Ed Maguire, who is the one person I miss the most. I don't miss my parents terribly, nor Kath, nor Paul (the real cutie I was going out with at summer's end), but I miss Edward a lot. But it's not terrible—there are so many wonderful people and things to do here that I can't miss anyone too much. All the same, I'll be glad to see him when he comes to visit on October 2.

It was wonderful to hear from you. I am all set to come visit you but the parental units have vetoed the idea, at least up to Winter Break. I'm working on them, but I think the 4-in-college has turned the trick. But I'm so tickled to be invited and it gives me something to think about and anticipate going to see Johnny in Sweden. Dave said winter is the time to go—with everything always lit up.

I've been writing between auditions but now I'm in my room with Annie, my suite mate—sweetmate. She's great. My auditions went OK—let me tell you about them:

The first was for the biggest, most professional theatre group, the Dramat. They're doing **Chicago** *and the audition was mostly dance. The* *steps were really hard but really fun. I was all worn out and sweating like a pig, and then they asked me to sing. I sang horribly but it was such fun. It got me in a great mood for my other auditions.*

The next was for **Once Upon A Mattress,** *by one of the move-the-chairs-in-the-dining room theatre groups. I sang horribly again but they asked me to read.*

Then I went to auditions for J.B., a straight show. That audition was fun too but they kept me waiting a long time and almost made me late for my next, last and best audition. The Yale Musical Theatre is doing Brecht's **Threepenny Opera.** *For the first time all evening, I sang well, both my fast song and my ballad. And they really liked the way I read. And they talked about hearing me sing from the score and practically* **told** *me I'd be called back. That's the show I'd really like to do, too.*

That's great that you're learning Swedish—you'll have to write me all those useful little expressions like, "hello," "thank you," and "two Swedish meatball, please." I already know how to say "Ja"

Love,
Steph

*　　　*　　　*

Daniel M. Singer
Washington, D.C.

September 6, 1981

Dear Judy and Mike –

Your letter reached us as we said "scoot" to our children, all of whom are at college. Dave & Steph at Yale and Amy & Ellen in Swarthmore. And Maxine and I celebrate with two weeks in France beginning next week. She has a meeting in Montpellier and I'm just stealing the time. By now you know that David was a good messenger for the Orrefors bowl—a lovely one it is.

Thanks much for your kind words about him. You two and John surely bring out the best in him and I know he loves all of you deeply.

From the tales told by Dave and William of their visit with John, we are convinced that John has some very special inner strength and enormous reservoir of whatever is required to look adversity in the eye and come away laughing.

We look forward to seeing for ourselves just how remarkable you and he have been.

Our love to all,

Dan

* * *

St. Albans School
Mount St. Alban
Washington, D.C.

Headmaster's Study

September 9, 1981

Dear John:

I have not yet had a report from Dave Singer or William Mondale, but I do hope they had a good visit with you and will come back with information about your continued improvement.

St. Albans is gearing up for the start of school. We began faculty meetings just before Labor Day and have the first day of classes on the 10th. Of course the football team has been hard at it for some time. This year we are going to be small and inexperienced, but the team seems to have very good spirit.

Do take care. Everyone here is thrilled when we have a good report about you.

Sincerely yours,

Mark H. Mullin
Headmaster

* * *

Kirk Mathews
United States Military Academy
West Point, New York

September 22, 1981

Dear John,

Hey! I know what you're saying. You can't believe I'd go to a hellhole like this, well, I did. I am playing football too. I am just kicking now 'cause I screwed my left knee up in wrestling and I had to have it operated on. I've been here for 84 days and haven't even come close to getting out in the civilian world. The work is really hard 'cause I take 20½ hours per week.

We lost to Missouri 24-10 and lost to VMI 14-7. We should've won both but we lost on careless errors. Anyway, we play Brown this weekend. I hope Mike comes up. Well I have to go and call my sister 'cause it is her birthday. Take care of those Swedish babes for me. (You think you could send me one special delivery?) Take it easy, bud.

Love,
Kirk

* * *

John Meehan
Utrecht, Holland

September 30, 1981

Dear John,

You don't know me, but I had the pleasure of getting to know a lot about you last year. My name is John, also, and I'm a good friend of Dave Singers at Yale. Last year I was a so-called "freshman counselor" (although they counseled us more than we counseled them) and I got to know Dave pretty well.

I graduated last May and am presently living in Utrecht, Holland. I did see Dave in early September and he gave me your address in Stockholm. I'm playing ice hockey here for a full season. Upon completion of the season, I plan on doing some traveling. Although I do not plan on seeing Sweden (again—I went on a hockey trip there once), but one never knows. At any rate, I'm extending an invitation to you to stop by here if you're ever passing through the area.

The reason I'm writing this letter is because I'm impressed with your strength and fight in dealing with your accident. Having an uncle who has been very sick for the last ten years, I understand what **real** *strength is. I hope things continue to go well for you.*

Sincerely,
John Meehan

* * *

Pete Hawley
Alexandria, Virginia

September 1981

Dear John,

How are you doing, Champ? Great, I hope. I don't know what I've been thinking, not writing to you, and I apologize.

Mom said that you were doing well and I'm really happy to hear it. She was ecstatic over how well you are doing. When do you get our new leg? Sorry if that's a sore subject. No pun intended. I know you. You must be sick of hearing how everybody feels sorry for you, and I know you don't need all that pity. Don't misunderstand this, but you're probably one of the best people for it to happen to because you're kind of tough O-O-O-O-N-N-N-N-CE in a while and can handle about anything.

School just started. There are a lot of good-looking girls in all my classes (except weightlifting.) I'll have to check 'em all out. We've got a mean team (expect to go to regionals.) Our defense held Hayfield to 14 total yards of offense, spear-headed by High School All American linebacker Carl Carr (6'3", 200 lbs., 4.3 sec 40 yds. Bench presses 325 lbs) I started at left tackle. We play 5 top 20 teams in Virginia (four in our district). Say hi to Joanne, and your Mom and Dad for me. Tell your Mom we sold the Vega, so I'm breathing easy for now. Write back soon.

Your friend,
Pete

*   *   *

St. Albans School
Mount St. Alban
Washington, D.C.

Headmaster's Study

October 5, 1981

Dear John:

It was great to have your letter, but I must say it did not contain any surprises. The fact that you are playing Frisbee, dancing, and dating a Swedish nurse is exactly what I would have expected of you, but it still cheers me immensely to have my predictions confirmed by the man himself.

It may be a long football season here. We lost to Bishop Ireton for the first time in many years and just squeaked by Wilson High School last week. Now we move into the IAC games. The team certainly has its work cut out for it. Soccer is a little better than last year but not nearly what it was in your time. Cross-country remains awesomely powerful as always.

The School has twelve new computers which are keeping the math buffs excited and Mr. Brown has had his lecture notes published. I must confess that I have not and will not read the book but it is an impressive collection of his fine work.

I'm so glad that you had some St. Albans visitors this summer. You know you have many friends here who continue to ask about you, as well as those of us who keep you in our prayers. Very best wishes, I know you have many people to write to but I am always cheered by your great letters.

Sincerely yours,

Mark H. Mullin
Headmaster

*　　　*　　　*

Bitsy Cronin
University of Alabama
Tuscaloosa, Alabama

October 19, 1981

Dear John,

What's happening???? Sorry I haven't written sooner but I've been so busy. How are the Swedish lessons going? That sounds really exciting and I'm really glad to hear that you're getting back into the school routine. I really can't wait until you can give me a few lessons.

School's going really well for a change, I like all my classes and I'm studying a lot more that I used to. I'm taking Special Education, Early Childhood Education, English, and French, of course. I guess I'm planning to major in it. I don't know, I really haven't decided but I like everything a lot and am putting a lot of effort into it.

I really haven't kept up with the Washington folks. I think that I'm slowly growing further and further away from it. It seems so strange because I remember making a promise to never to lose touch with our friends from Buckles' Basement, Class of '80, etc. But I've only been in D.C. for three weeks this year, working at camp and all, and I haven't even seen Jenny since May!! I called Jud when I was home after camp (three days) but he never called me back. Its like I have a whole different set of friends. Let's you and I keep in touch though, OK?

Well John, let me know how things are going. I think about you very often. Take care and say "hey" to your family for me.

Lots of love,
Bitsy

* * *

Billy Mondale
Brown University
Providence, Rhode Island

October 26, 1981

Dear John,

How's Uppsala? May have notice, my organization has been lax. Lax has been kind of lax, too now that I think of it. Basically Brown has been treating me very well; I'm back in love again with Francene (you know, my girl from last year), I'm enjoying the fraternity, my school work while not (ever) being good enough is going along, i.e. I'm studying & going to classes and liking both. Besides, the library is the best place to pick up girls.

I'm taking a course in Impressionism, which is really super. I'm reading Machiavelli for my history course, and think about old Beegles and Davis when I learn the stuff. Malones and I are getting along fine and the room is hot, too. My sister says hello. She's really having some troubles but I hope she'll pull through. She's both strong and weak at the same time.

How's Isabelle? Say hello, and to your wonderful family. By the way, you should write sometime, but look at me, it took a whole month for me!! I'm thinking about learning squash. Are you playing? How's Swedish (Svedish)? Take care, stay in touch.

Love,
Billy

* * *

Mary Cronin
Bethesda, Maryland

December 1, 1981

Dear John,

How thoughtful to remember us on your trip to Germany. We appreciated your thoughts of keeping us up to date. Don and I visited Garmish many years ago and I remember it as a Brigadoon—something of a paradise lost in the shuffle of a new world. You may remember the painting over our sofa in the living room; we bought it in Garmish.

I'd like for you to know how much we missed you on Thanksgiving Day! Bee did not come home either, so Dan and I had a quiet day alone. For the life of me, I will never adjust to Bee's absence. I'm certain she has written all about her roommate problems. In this regard, she has not been successful. In spite of her trauma, she is making good grades. Would you believe some A's?? She has pretty definitely decided to major in French. Quite truthfully, I am delighted with her choice so I hope there isn't a further change. She loves being at the University of Alabama, however, and being a Southern Girl! Sometime long into the future, Don and I will return to Alabama. We would like to buy a home at Point Clear, right on the water. Until then, we'll just have to make occasional trips to our condo on the Gulf. It is quite lovely and I do want you to go down with us for a visit when you get home.

I manage to see Suzy but not as often now that she is back at school. We did meet in Georgetown this past Saturday for lunch. Did I ever tell you that her college roommate is the wife of one of Don's best friends in Alabama? This is a small world! John, you will love the new Georgetown Park—so many shops—all first class. We'll take you there. Also, there's a new shop call the Hat Belfry—knowing your love for hats, you'll have a wild time in this shop.

I wish I had news of your friends. Only when Bee is home do I hear the goings-on. Many called here during Thanksgiving so I did chat with a few but they suppress the news to me. I'm sure she will bring you up to date when she gets home which should be about Dec. 15. We'll be here til Dec. 27 and then will go to Nassau for eight days. We're all feeling the need for a rest. Mine and Don's vacation was spent cleaning the condo. Bee will have to leave a couple of days after we get back so her time at home will be short.

Fat Liz sends her paw-paw greetings to you. Honestly, she is aging fast. Don thinks she is older than the eight years we set for her.

John, we wish you a cheery, fun-filled Christmas and New Years. I told your parents we will keep Champagne on ice til you return and your return in 1982 will make the New Year an exciting one for all of us!

Joy and love to our John from,
Mary, Don, and Liz

* * *

Mrs. John W. Cole
Randolph, Vermont

December 16, 1981

Dear Judy,

Sadie called us to tell us about John's terrible accident but she was so upset, we didn't have too clear an idea what had happened. Later Ruth Johnson had been visiting Phil and sent us your letter to him about what had happened. We hope John is continuing to recover satisfactorily. You and Mike have certainly had more than your share of trouble. I hope there is an end to it now and all your family have a safe and happy life from now on.

We count ourselves most fortunate to have had so few problems among the Coles. We now have five great grandchildren—all Boyd & Betty's grandchildren.

The boy Ann was living with since her divorce has moved out for which we are all grateful. She is much happier and has found a new friend who lives in Hanover. Ann still has her little house in White River. We plan to go to Connecticut to our son John's for Christmas.

John has stopped competitive shooting so we didn't go to Demariscotta this year. He has early cataracts and glaucoma in both eyes. I have the same but only in the right eye. The doctor claims most everyone has one or both problems when they reach 70. We are both guilty of that.

Our life in Vermont continues to be enjoyable. We play golf in the summer—poorly. John skis a little at Stowe in the winter. He has a lifetime free pass there. They give them to anyone over 70.

When you get back to this country, I hope you can come see us. We would love to have you, summer or winter.

Love to you and all your family,

Susie

Index

Index of Letter Writers

Glossary of Terms:

AAIRA: Assistant Air Attaché
AALUSNA: Assistant Naval Attaché
AIRA: Air Attaché
ALUSNA: Naval Attaché
ARMA: Army Attaché
CINC: Commander in Chief
DAO: Defense Attaché Office
DATT: Defense Attaché
DIA: Defense Intelligence Agency
Fo/INT: Defense International Office
FRG: Federal Republic of Germany
FSI: Foreign Service Institute
NCS: National Cathedral School (Girls)
PAS: Professor of Aerospace Science
STA: St. Albans School
STK: Stockholm
UNH: University of New Hampshire
USMA: United States Military Academy

www.ingramcontent.com/pod-product-compliance
Lightning Source LLC
Chambersburg PA
CBHW061335280526
45784CB00001B/23
* 9 7 8 0 5 9 5 1 5 2 2 4 7 *